Diabetic Gourmet Cookbook

• • •

Mary Jane Finsand

Foreword by
James D. Healy, M.D., F.A.A.P.

Sterling Publishing Co., Inc. **New York**
Blandford Press   Dorset, England

Library of Congress Cataloging-in-Publication Data

Finsand, Mary Jane.
  Diabetic gourmet cookbook.

  Includes index.
  1. Diabetes—Diet therapy—Recipes.   I. Title.
  RC662.F5656 1986   641.5'6314   86-14354
  ISBN 0-8069-6372-7
  ISBN 0-8069-6374-3 (pbk.)

3   5   7   9   10   8   6   4   2

Copyright © 1986 by Mary Jane Finsand
Published by Sterling Publishing Co., Inc.
Two Park Avenue, New York, N.Y. 10016
Distributed in Canada by Oak Tree Press Ltd.
% Canadian Manda Group, P.O. Box 920, Station U
Toronto, Ontario, Canada M8Z 5P9
Distributed in the United Kingdom by Blandford Press
Link House, West Street, Poole, Dorset BH15 1LL, England
Distributed in Australia by Capricorn Ltd.
P.O. Box 665, Lane Cove, NSW 2066
Manufactured in the United States of America
All rights reserved

Contents

Foreword

Users of Mary Jane Finsand's four other diabetic cookbooks know that diabetics can eat a wide variety of delicious foods and still follow a doctor prescribed diabetic diet. Adding gourmet variety to an already restricted diet can appear to be a difficult problem. With the *Diabetic Gourmet Cookbook,* Mary Jane has created recipes for scrumptious foods that will really tempt a gourmet's palate. This cookbook will help diabetics and other people on restricted diets.

Each recipe in this cookbook includes calorie and food exchange information for each serving. This completeness allows diabetics and other readers to regulate food intake within medically prescribed recommendations while eating gourmet-style foods.

Although written specifically for the diabetic, this cookbook is an excellent reference for anyone interested in eating balanced gourmet foods and meals. Please share this cookbook with your own doctor, pharmacy, hospital dietician, and diabetic organization. I am confident that they will confirm my high recommendation.

James D. Healy, M.D., F.A.A.P.

A Note from Schoitz
Diabetes Education Resource Center

The *Diabetic Gourmet Cookbook* is a must for all diabetics interested in food that is different in taste. The recipes are not just for diabetics on the exchange diet; calculations are included for diabetics and other people who are on the carbohydrate system. Many of your friends who are not diabetics will also enjoy these gourmet recipes. Include these recipes in your menu planning, especially for social or family functions, to add flexibility and variety.

If you have any questions concerning your diet, please feel free to contact us.

Hattie M. Middleton, R.D., diabetes educator
Darlene Duke, R.N., diabetes educator
Schoitz Diabetes Education Resource Center
2101 Kimball Avenue
Waterloo, IA 50702

Introduction

I knew it would not take long before you—my diabetic readers—would want the finest of foods. If you are either on the exchange diet or the carbohydrate diet, you must limit the amount of food you eat. And, of course, you want that food to be the best. So why not cook gourmet dishes?

For too many people, the word "gourmet" evokes images of long hours and tedious food preparation. But it really means a person who is fond of and can appreciate fine foods and drinks. My mother, who was known for her fine cooking, would proclaim: "Being a gourmet cook is nothing more than learning to cook what your neighbors cook." And so, we ate the finest—from oysters on the half-shell to chateaubriand, from German torte to apple pandowdy.

I owe both my inspiration and knowledge to write this book to my mother. I dedicate this book to her. For it was through her that I acquired interest in gourmet foods—wonderful ethnic foods from all over the world and marvellous regional dishes from all over the United States.

Because I have already written the *Diabetic Candy, Cookie & Dessert Cookbook* (Sterling Publishing Co., Inc., 1982) and *The Diabetic Chocolate Cookbook* (Sterling Publishing Co., Inc., 1984), I felt I would use most of this cookbook for recipes other than desserts. But I am sure that you can find just about anything you like for dessert in any of my other cookbooks.

My aim in writing this book is to provide knowlege in both food terms and food that is the best of the finest.

Bon appétit.

Mary Jane Finsand

Using the Recipes

Read the recipes carefully. Then assemble all equipment and ingredients. Use standard measuring equipment (whether metric or customary); be sure to measure accurately.

Remember, these recipes are good for *everyone*, not just the diabetic. All liquids—milk, water etc.—used in recipes are *cold* unless otherwise noted. All recipes found in this book are capitalized. Check the index for page numbers when specific recipes call for recipes, such as Chateaubriand Sauce or Chicken Stock or Red Currant Jelly.

CONVERSION GUIDES

Customary Terms		Metric Symbols	
t.	teaspoon	mL	millilitre
T.	tablespoon	L	litre
c.	cup	g	gram
env.	envelope	kg	kilogram
pkg.	package	°C	degrees Celsius
pt.	pint	mm	millimetre
qt.	quart	cm	centimetre
oz.	ounce		
lb.	pound		
°F	degrees Fahrenheit		
in.	inch		

Cooking Pans and Casseroles

CUSTOMARY	METRIC
1 qt.	1 L
2 qt.	2 L
3 qt.	3 L

Guide to Approximate Equivalents

CUSTOMARY				METRIC	
Ounces Pounds	Cups	Tablespoons	Teaspoons	Millilitres	Grams Kilograms
			¼ t.	1 mL	1 g
			½ t.	2 mL	
			1 t.	5 mL	
			2 t.	10 mL	
½ oz.		1 T.	3 t.	15 mL	15 g
1 oz.		2 T.	6 t.	30 mL	30 g
2 oz.	¼ c.	4 T.	12 t.	60 mL	
4 oz.	½ c.	8 T.	24 t.	125 mL	
8 oz.	1 c.	16 T.	48 t.	250 mL	
2.2 lb.					1 kg
	4 c.			1 L	

Keep in mind that this is not an exact conversion, but generally may be used for food measurement. Also, some weights (ounces and grams) taken from manufacturers' packages may not be consistent or standard.

Guide to Pan Sizes

CUSTOMARY	HOLDS	METRIC	HOLDS
8-in. pie	2 c.	20-cm pie	600 mL
9-in. pie	1 qt.	23-cm pie	1 L
10-in. pie	1¼ qt.	25-cm pie	1.3 L
8-in. round	1 qt.	20-cm round	1 L
9-in. round	1½ qt.	23-cm round	1.5 L
8-in. square	2 qt.	20-cm square	2 L
9-in. square	2½ qt.	23-cm square	2.5 L
9×5×2-in. (loaf)	2 qt.	23×13×5-cm (loaf)	2 L
9-in. tube	3 qt.	23-cm tube	3 L
10-in. tube	3 qt.	25-cm tube	3 L
10-in. Bundt	3 qt.	25-cm Bundt	3 L
9×5 in.	1½ qt.	23×13 cm	1.5 L
10×6 in.	3½ qt.	25×16 cm	3.5 L
11×7 in.	3½ qt.	27×17 cm	3.5 L
13×9×2 in.	3½ qt.	33×23×5 cm	3.5 L
14×10 in.	cookie tin	36×25 cm	
15½×10½×1 in.	jelly roll	39×25×3 cm	

Oven Cooking Guides

FAHRENHEIT	OVEN HEAT	CELSIUS
°F		°C
250–275°	very slow	120–135°
300–325°	slow	150–165°
350–375°	moderate	175–190°
400–425°	hot	200–220°
450–475°	very hot	230–245°
475–500°	hottest	250–290°

Equivalent Food and Cookery Terms

AMERICAN	BRITISH
all-purpose flour	plain flour
bacon	rashers
broil	grill
brown sugar	demerara sugar
candy	sweets; confections
confectioners' (powdered) sugar	icing sugar
cookie	biscuit
cornstarch	cornflour
eggplant	aubergine
fine granulated white sugar	caster (castor) sugar
ground meat	minced meat
heavy cream	double cream
light cream	single cream
molasses	treacle
rock candy	rock sugar
scallion	spring or green onion
shrimp	prawn
squid (calamari)	inkfish
zucchini	baby marrow or courgette

Spices and Herbs

The word "spice" is usually defined as a group of aromatic plants grown in the tropics. Spices are made from various parts of the plant, most often not from the seeds or the leaves. For instance, clove is derived from the dried flower bud, black pepper from a dried berry, red pepper, ground chili pepper and allspice from dried fruit, ginger from the root, and cinnamon from the bark.

An "herb" owes its flavoring qualities to the soluble oil in the plants, leaves, or seeds. The herbs most widely used include basil, chive, dill, fennel, marjoram, oregano, parsley, sage, savory, tarragon, and thyme. But we should, also, think of using flowers as flavoring agents, such as the geranium, lavender, marigold, rose, and violet.

Some of the familiar products you find on your spice shelf are very powerful and could take over the flavor of the entire dish. After you have developed your personal taste for the spice or herb, then you may add as you like.

As a rule of thumb: ½ t. (2 mL) of a dried herb is equal to 1 T. (15 mL) of a fresh herb. Always crumble dried herbs before using them to release their flavor.

Hopefully, the following definitions will broaden your knowledge of herbs and spices as to their aromas, flavors, and also other characteristics, and at the same time encourage you to use them.

Allspice (a berry) has a flavor similar to a mixture of cinnamon, ginger, and nutmeg. Allspice is used in breads, pastries, jellies, jams, pickles, vegetable dishes, pork and sausage recipes.

Aniseed provides the licorice flavoring in candies, breads, fruit dishes, wine and liqueurs, as well as chicken dishes.

Basil (an herb leaf) has a sweet and strong flavor. It is used in Italian and Mediterranean-style cooking, such as meat, cheese, egg, and tomato dishes. Basil is easily grown in a garden or on a windowsill.

Bay leaf (often called sweet bay or laurel) is sweet but has a strong flavor. Use it with care as it can overpower foods. It is, however, excellent in stews or meat dishes, and in small amounts in any tomato dishes.

Celery has a pleasantly bitter flavor. Use celery in anything that is not sweet.

Chive provides a light onion flavor in anything you want. It adds lovely green color to bland-looking dishes.

Cinnamon (bark of the cassis cinnamon tree) has a pungent and sweet flavor. Use it in pastries, breads, pickles, wine, beer, and liqueurs.

Clove (bud of the clove tree) has a pungent and sweet flavor. Use whole cloves to stud hams and other meat products. Ground cloves are used in sauces, pastries, puddings, fruit dishes, wine, and liqueurs. Again, use it with care.

Marjoram leaves have a sweet, semi-pungent flavor. Marjoram is used in poultry, lamb, egg, and vegetable dishes.

Nutmeg and mace: Mace is the lacy skin of the nutmeg seed. Mace has a stronger flavor than nutmeg but these two spices can be used interchangeably in cooking. They both have spicy, sweet, nutty flavors. If I were to be accused of using any one spice too often, it would be nutmeg. I sprinkle a little on almost everything. Nutmeg can add a subtle, exciting flavor to meats, sauces, vegetables, and particularly, desserts.

Oregano leaves have a sweet, pungent flavor. Oregano is used in meat, pasta, and vegetable dishes. Dried oregano is always available. I can usually find fresh oregano in shops near my home and enjoy using it.

Parsley has a bright green leaf with a fresh clean flavor. Parsley can be seen garnishing plates from truck stops to the finest restaurants. Its flavor blends well with all other seasonings and can stand on its own. Although I am not including many common herbs and spices, I feel I should include parsley in this list. I like to consider parsley as a true American herb (even though the French also use it extensively).

Paprika, one of the chilies, has a sweet flavor. It is used in salads, vegetables, poultry, fish, and egg dishes. Paprika is often used as a color garnish.

Pepper (a berry): Black Pepper is produced when the pepper berry is picked before it ripens and dries. It wrinkles and turns black. White pepper is produced when the pepper berry is allowed to ripen before picking. The outer shell is removed to expose the white core. White pepper is milder and sweeter than black pepper.

Rosemary (a leaf) has a sweet, fresh, woody flavor similar to pine needles. Use rosemary in soup, meat, and vegetable dishes. Experiment with flavor before adding rosemary in large quantities.

Sage (a leaf) has a pungent, bitter flavor. I suggest using sage for stuffings, sausages, and other meat dishes. Try a small amount in vegetables and soups. Sage is easily grown in a garden or a flowerpot.

Thyme (a leaf) has a pungent, semibitter flavor. Thyme adds flavor to many dishes. But use it sparingly.

Beverages

I am placing beverages first in this cookbook for a very good reason. At almost every function or gathering you are greeted with something to drink. The word "beverage" derives from the Latin word *bibere*, which means "to drink." According to standard dictionaries, beverages are all liquids for drinking, such as milk, coffee, tea, fruit drinks, or alcoholic drinks.

In a gourmet cookbook, I believe the presentation of all drinks to your guests is important and sets the mood of the occasion. At a formal dinner, for example, you might add a thin slice of lemon, lime, or orange to the water glass: A fruit slice keeps the water tasting fresher and also offers a sense of elegance. A small piece or fruit, such as a strawberry or peach slice, is particularly nice when served in a glass of white wine or champagne.

Ice moulds are delightful to serve in your beverages. When making an ice mould, rinse the mould with water; then place the mould in a freezer. When chilled, add a few pieces of garnish, such as thin slices of fruit or washed, fresh leaves and put back into the freezer. Make your nonalcoholic punch mixture into a slush. (To make a slush, place container in freezer until partially frozen.) Pour slush into the chilled mould and allow the punch to freeze. (Alcohol doesn't freeze well.) If you are using ice cubes or crushed ice in your punch, float thin slices of fruit or leaves on top. When ready to serve, set your punch bowl on a tray to eliminate the possibility of punch stains on your tablecloth.

Hot beverages should always be kept hot. I know this sounds silly, but I have received many lukewarm cups of coffee because the cups were filled at the coffee service rather than brought to the table. You don't need a silver service to serve a hot beverage at the table. A cute, inexpensive teapot will work just fine. For a buffet, serve your hot beverage as the last item on the table.

Brisk Punch

This punch is great for any kind of party where you do not want to serve alcohol.

1 pkg.	low-calorie drink mix	1 pkg.
2 c.	cold water	500 mL
1 qt.	salt-free seltzer or sparkling water	1 L

Combine the drink mix and cold water; stir to dissolve mix. At serving time, add the seltzer. Pour over ice in glasses or place the ice or an ice mould in a punch bowl and add the punch.

Yield: 10 servings
Exchange, 1 serving: negligible
Calories, 1 serving: negligible
Carbohydrates, 1 serving: negligible

Juice Punch

2 qts.	low-calorie cranberry juice cocktail	2 L
2 c.	orange juice	500 mL
3 T.	lemon juice, freshly squeezed	45 mL
1 qt.	water	1 L
2 qts.	sugar-free tonic water	2 L

Combine the juices and water; stir to blend. Chill thoroughly. Just before serving, add the tonic water. Serve over ice in glasses or place the ice or an ice mould in a punch bowl and add the punch.

Yield: 36 servings
Exchange, 1 serving: ½ fruit
Calories, 1 serving: 16
Carbohydrates, 1 serving: 4 g

Spicy Cranberry Punch with Champagne

1 recipe	Spicy Cranberry Punch (without the seltzer or sparkling water)	1 recipe
1½ qts.	champagne	1.5 L
5	lemon slices, thinly sliced	5

Proceed as directed in Spicy Cranberry Punch. Pour the champagne into the punch instead of the seltzer. Serve in a punch bowl and float the lemon slices on top.

Yield: 25 servings
Exchange, 1 serving: 2 fruit
Calories, 1 serving: 81
Carbohydrates, 1 serving: 20 g

Apricot-Pineapple Punch

1½ c.	apricot nectar	375 mL
1½ c.	pineapple juice	375 mL
¾ c.	orange juice concentrate, frozen	190 mL
1 c.	water	250 mL
½ c.	lemon juice	125 mL
4	bananas, mashed	4
4 qts.	sugar-free ginger ale	4 L

Combine the juices, concentrate, water, and bananas; stir to blend. Refrigerate until thoroughly chilled. Just before serving, add the ginger ale. Serve over ice in glasses or place the ice or an ice mould in a punch bowl and add the punch.

Yield: 30 servings
Exchange, 1 serving: 1 fruit
Calories, 1 serving: 39
Carbohydrates, 1 serving: 10 g

Apricot-Pineapple Sauterne Punch

1 recipe	Apricot-Pineapple Punch (without the ginger ale)	1 recipe
⁴/₅ qt.	sauterne	.75 L
5	lemon slices, thinly sliced	5
6	orange slices, thinly sliced	6
	mint leaves for garnish	

Proceed as directed in Apricot-Pineapple Punch. Pour the sauterne into the punch instead of the ginger ale. Serve in a punch bowl and float the lemon and orange slices and mint leaves on top.

Yield: 19 servings
Exchange, 1 serving: 2½ fruit
Calories, 1 serving: 95
Carbohydrates, 1 serving: 24 g

Spicy Cranberry Punch

16-oz. can	cranberry gel	454-g can
1 qt.	water	1 L
4 pkg.	Equal low-calorie sweetener	4 pkg.
¼ c.	lemon juice	60 mL
½ t.	ground or grated nutmeg	2 mL
1 qt.	salt-free seltzer or sparkling water	1 L

Melt the cranberry gel in a saucepan. Stir in the water, lemon juice, and nutmeg. Bring to the boil; boil 2 minutes. Remove from heat and cool to room temperature. Stir in the sweetener. Allow to mellow for 3 to 4 days in the refrigerator. Just before serving, add the seltzer. Serve over ice in glasses or place the ice or an ice mould in a punch bowl and add the punch.

Yield: 20 servings
Exchange, 1 serving: 1 fruit
Calories, 1 serving: 41
Carbohydrates, 1 serving: 11 g

Orange Sherbet Cooler

4 qts.	orange sherbet	4 L
3 qts.	sugar-free tonic water	3 L

Place sherbet in a punch bowl. Pour tonic water over the sherbet. Serve immediately.

Yield: 38 servings
Exchange, 1 serving: 1 bread
*   1 fruit*
Calories, 1 serving: 114
Carbohydrates, 1 serving: 24 g

Summer Russian Tea

A lovely cooler for luncheon on a hot day.

2 c.	sugar-free orange breakfast drink mix	500 mL
½ c.	instant tea	125 mL
1 pkg.	sugar-free lemonade drink mix	1 pkg.
2 t.	ground cinnamon	10 mL
1 t.	ground cloves	5 mL

Combine all ingredients in a glass jar; shake to blend. To serve, place 1 T. (15 mL) of the mix in a large iced tea glass and fill two-thirds full with cold water; stir to dissolve mixture. Add ice.

Yield: 18 servings
Exchange, 1 serving: negligible
Calories, 1 serving: 4
Carbohydrates, 1 serving: 1 g

Tomato Cocktail

1 qt. 14-oz. can	tomato juice	1.36-L can
1	cucumber, peeled and grated	1
3	green onions, finely chopped	3
3 T.	lemon juice, freshly squeezed	45 mL
1 T.	Worcestershire sauce	15 mL
1 T.	fresh horseradish, grated	15 mL
dash of each	salt, pepper, and Tabasco sauce	dash of each

Combine all ingredients in a large glass container; mix thoroughly. Refrigerate until chilled. Strain. Serve chilled.

Yield: 10 servings
Exchange, 1 serving: 1 vegetable
Calories, 1 serving: 28
Carbohydrates, 1 serving: 6 g

"Apmato" Appetizer Cocktail

2 c.	apple juice	500 mL
2 c.	tomato juice	500 mL
1 T.	lemon juice, freshly squeezed	15 mL
6	whole cloves	6
½ t.	Dijon-style mustard	2 mL
¼ t.	fresh basil leaves, whole or minced	1 mL

Combine all ingredients in a saucepan. Bring just to the boil; reduce heat and simmer for 3 minutes. Strain. Serve hot.

Yield: 12 servings
Exchange, 1 serving: 1 vegetable
Calories, 1 serving: 27
Carbohydrates, 1 serving: 5 g

Hot Autumn Punch

. . . with the taste of cinnamon and cloves

2 qts.	black tea	2 L
1½ qts.	low-calorie cranberry juice cocktail	1½ L
1½ qts.	apple juice	1½ L
3 c.	orange juice	750 mL
½ c.	lemon juice	125 mL
⅓ c.	granulated sugar replacement	90 mL
6	cinnamon sticks, broken	6
18	whole cloves	18

Combine all ingredients in a large saucepan. Bring to the boil, reduce heat and simmer for 5 minutes. Strain. Serve hot.

Yield: 36 servings
Exchange, 1 serving: 1 fruit
Calories, 1 serving: 45
Carbohydrates, 1 serving: 11 g

Clam Juice Cocktail

6 c.	clam juice	1.5 L
¼ c.	celery with leaves, chopped	60 mL
¼ c.	fresh parsley, chopped	60 mL
2	garlic cloves, chopped	2
	fresh lemon juice	

Combine all ingredients in a saucepan. Bring to the boil; reduce heat and simmer for 4 minutes. Strain well. Ladle into hot cups and sprinkle with the desired amount of lemon juice.

Yield: 12 servings
Exchange, 1 serving: ½ vegetable
Calories, 1 serving: 11
Carbohydrates, 1 serving: 2 g

Wedding Punch

1 t.	ground nutmeg	5 mL
2 c.	strong black tea, hot	500 mL
1½ qts.	low-calorie cranberry juice cocktail	1½ L
6-oz. can	lemonade, frozen	177-g can
1 qt.	diet lemon-lime soda	1 L

Stir the nutmeg into the hot tea. Cool to room temperature. Add the cranberry cocktail and lemonade; stir to thaw lemonade. Refrigerate until chilled. Just before serving, add the soda. Pour over ice in glasses or place the ice or an ice mould into a punch bowl and add the punch.

Yield: 20 servings
Exchange, 1 serving: 1 fruit
Calories, 1 serving: 35
Carbohydrates, 1 serving: 9 g

Orange Blossom Punch

6 c.	*orange juice*	*1.5 L*
1 pkg.	*low-calorie orange-drink mix*	*1 pkg.*
1 qt.	*water*	*1 L*
2 c.	*vodka*	*500 mL*
2 qts.	*salt-free seltzer*	*2 L*
	orange slices for garnish	
	lemon slices for garnish	
	mint leaves for garnish	

Combine the juice, drink mix, and water in a large bowl; stir to dissolve the mix. Add the vodka. Just before serving, pour the punch over crushed ice. Add the seltzer. Garnish with fruit slices and mint leaves.

Yield: 32
Exchange, 1 serving: ½ fruit
Calories, 1 serving: 23
Carbohydrates, 1 serving: 5 g

Fruit-of-the-Vine Punch

1 qt.	*grape juice*	*1 L*
1 qt.	*white grape juice*	*1 L*
1 qt.	*white wine (preferably Rhine)*	*1 L*
1 qt.	*salt-free seltzer*	*1 L*

Combine all the ingredients. Pour over ice or an ice mould in a punch bowl. Serve immediately. (The punch may be garnished with grapes and/ or lemon slices.)

Yield: 26 servings
Exchange, 1 serving: 2 fruit
Calories, 1 serving: 80
Carbohydrates, 1 serving: 14 g

Orange Nog

6	egg yolks	6
6-oz. can	orange juice concentrate, thawed	177-g can
¼ c.	lemon juice, freshly squeezed	60 mL
1 t.	ground nutmeg	5 mL
5 c.	skim milk	1.25 L
6	egg whites, beaten stiff	6

Beat the egg yolks until foamy. Slowly add the orange juice concentrate, lemon juice, and nutmeg. Beat in the milk. Gently fold in the egg whites. Serve in Irish coffee mugs.

Yield: 12 servings
Exchange, 1 serving: 1 nonfat milk
⅓ fruit
Calories, 1 serving: 103
Carbohydrates, 1 serving: 14 g

Port Punch

3 c.	orange juice	750 mL
1½ c.	lemon juice, freshly squeezed	375 mL
1½ c.	port	375 mL
½ t.	ground or grated nutmeg	2 mL
⅛ t.	ground ginger	.5 mL
5 c.	diet lemon-lime soda	1.25 L

Combine juices, port, and spices in a glass jar. Cover and refrigerate; allow the mixture to mellow for 3 to 4 days. Strain. Just before serving, pour over ice or an ice mould in a punch bowl. Add the soda.

Yield: 30 servings
Exchange, 1 serving: ⅔ fruit
Calories, 1 serving: 26
Carbohydrates, 1 serving: 4 g

Jamaican Rum Punch

2 c.	orange juice	500 mL
¾ c.	lemon juice, freshly squeezed	190 mL
3 c.	white rum	750 mL

1	cinnamon stick, broken	1
5½ c.	sugar-free ginger ale	1.38 L
	orange slices	

Combine the juices, rum, and cinnamon stick in a glass jar. Cover and refrigerate; allow the mixture to mellow for 4 to 5 days. Strain. Just before serving, pour over ice. Add the ginger ale. Garnish with the orange slices. (This punch is prettier if crushed ice or ice cubes are used rather than an ice mould.)

Yield: 30 servings
Exchange, 1 serving: 1½ fruit
Calories, 1 serving: 59
Carbohydrates, 1 serving: 14 g

Peach Cordial

10 lbs.	fresh peaches	4.6 kg
6 c.	water	1.5 L
1	cinnamon stick, broken	1
1	whole ground or grated nutmeg	1
2 t.	whole cloves	10 mL
½ t.	ground allspice	2 mL
3 env.	aspartame sweetener	3 env.
½ c.	liquid fructose	125 mL
1 qt.	brandy	1 L

Peel, pit, and dice the peaches. Combine the peaches and water in a saucepan. Bring to the boil; reduce heat, cover, and simmer for an hour. Strain through 3 layers of cheesecloth spread in a large strainer. Extract as much liquid as possible. You should have about 2 qts. (2 L) of nectar; if not, add enough water to make 2 qts. (2 L). Combine the nectar and spices in a saucepan. Heat to the boiling point; reduce heat, cover, and simmer for 20 minutes. Remove from heat and cool to room temperature. Add the sweeteners and stir to blend. Stir in the brandy. Pour into sterilized glass bottles and cover tightly. Allow the mixture to mellow in a dark, dry place for 3 weeks. Decant the clear liquid, discarding any sediment. Rebottle and store for 2 to 3 months before serving.

Yield: 30 servings
Exchange, 1 serving: 2 fruit
Calories, 1 serving: 76
Carbohydrates, 1 serving: 19 g

Warm Wine Dessert Drink

¾ c.	water	190 mL
2	cinnamon sticks, broken	2
½	lemon, cut in small chucks	½
24	whole cloves	24
1 qt.	pineapple juice	1 L
½ c.	granulated sugar replacement	125 mL
1 qt.	pink champagne	1 L

Boil the water with the cinnamon, lemon chunks, and cloves for 5 minutes; cool slightly. Add the pineapple juice and sugar replacement and heat slightly. Stir in the champagne and heat just to warm the mixture; strain. Serve warm, garnished with lemon slices.

Yield: 20 servings
Exchange, 1 serving: 1¾ fruit
Calories, 1 serving: 66
Carbohydrates, 1 serving: 16 g

Royal Rum Cocktail

6 bags	black tea	6 bags
1 qt.	boiling water	1 L
1	cinnamon stick, broken	1
2 to 3	lemon slices	2 to 3
1 c.	dark rum	250 mL
1 qt.	diet cola, chilled	1 L

Place the tea bags, cinnamon pieces, and lemon slices in a heatproof pitcher. Pour in the boiling water; steep for 20 minutes. Refrigerate until chilled. Strain. Just before serving, add the rum and cola. Serve chilled in champagne glasses.

Yield: 14 servings
Exchange, 1 serving: 1 fruit
Calories, 1 serving: 36
Carbohydrates, 1 serving: 9 g

Mint Julep

1 T.	water	15 mL
½ t.	granulated sugar replacement	2 mL
3	mint leaves	3
1½ oz.	bourbon	45 g

Place water, sugar replacement, and mint leaves in a mortar. Pound with a pestle until well mashed and blended. Pour into a frosted glass filled with crushed ice. Stir in the bourbon. If desired, garnish with mint leaves and a short drinking straw (the straw is to keep your nose out of the strongly scented mint leaves).

Yield: 1 serving
Exchange: 2 fruit
Calories: 82
Carbohydrates: 20 g

Sizzling Summer Refresher

¾ c.	orange juice	190 mL
¼ c.	salt-free seltzer or sparkling water	60 mL
1 T.	vodka	15 mL

Fill a tall goblet with ice cubes. Pour in all the ingredients and stir to mix.

Yield: 1 serving
Exchange: 2 fruit
Calories: 82
Carbohydrates: 19 g

Appetizers

Appetizers provide for you the opportunity to create food that is attractive in both shape and color. Appetizers can be hot or cold, can range from a simple dip to an elaborate rolled sandwich. You can combine interesting flavors and textures.

Since they are meant to stimulate the appetite, appetizers should be served in small portions. An appetizer should never be in the same food family as the main course. For instance, if you are serving fish for the main course, don't serve a shrimp cocktail as the appetizer.

Every nationality can boast appetizers: The Scandinavians have a smorgasbord, Italians an antipasto, French the canapés and hors d'oeuvres, and Americans the dips, dunks, and nibbles. The various names specify the type or kind of appetizer. Here are some examples:

Canapé—a dainty open-faced sandwich. Canapés, either hot or cold, can be served on bread, crackers, or some type of pastry base.

Cocktail—one or a group of vegetables, fruits, or seafoods served cold with a sauce. Cocktails are usually served at the table, such as shrimp cocktail.

Dips and dunks—hot or cold creamy mixtures, which are scooped up on a vegetable section, potato or corn chip, or cracker.

Hors d'oeuvre—a hot or cold appetizer, usually served at the table and eaten with a knife and fork. Unlike canapés, hors d'oeuvres do not have a pastry or bread base.

Nibbles—any food that can be picked up by a small fork, toothpick, or fingers. The varied collection of nibbles includes cheese or meat cubes, nuts, and olives.

Relishes—a variety of vegetables.

Spreads—similiar to dips, but firm enough to be spread on a pastry base.

I admit I like appetizers. The small portions allow me to eat small amounts of many different flavors and types of foods. On several occasions, I have served only appetizers as the entire meal.

Spreads

I would feel remiss if I did not adapt this recipe for you from *The Complete Diabetic Cookbook* (Sterling Publishing Co. Inc., 1980). So many of you have told me how much you enjoy these spreads.

Yield: ¼ c. (60 mL) spread for 24 crackers or ½ t. (2 mL) per cracker.
Exchange per serving: ½ fat plus cracker exchange

Use one of the following recipes as a spread for 24 crackers.

Anchovy

| 1 oz. | anchovy fillets | 30 g |
| ¼ c. | low-calorie margarine | 60 mL |

Rinse the fillets in cold water; pat dry. Grind or chop finely; blend with the margarine. Allow to rest.

Exchange, ¼ c. (60 mL): 12 fat
Calories, ¼ c. (60 mL): 250
Carbohydrates, ¼ c. (60 mL): negligible

Herb

| dash of each | marjoram, oregano, onion, finely chopped, salt, and pepper | dash of each |
| ¼ c. | low-calorie margarine | 60 mL |

Exchange, ¼ c. (60 mL): 12 fat
Calories, ¼ c. (60 mL): 200
Carbohydrates, ¼ c. (60 mL): negligible

Horseradish

1 T.	horseradish, grated	15 mL
1 t.	parsley, chopped	5 mL
¼ c.	low-calorie margarine	60 mL

Blend ingredients together; refrigerate overnight.

Exchange, ¼ c. (60 mL): 12 fat
Calories, ¼ c. (60 mL): 200
Carbohydrates, ¼ c. (60 mL): negligible

Caviar

| 2 T. | caviar | 30 mL |
| ¼ c. | low-calorie margarine | 60 mL |

Combine the caviar and margarine. Refrigerate overnight.

Exchange, ¼ c. (60 mL): 12 fat
Calories, ¼ c. (60 mL): 280
Carbohydrates, ¼ c. (60 mL): negligible

Crab Meat

| 2 T. | crab meat | 30 mL |
| ¼ c. | low-calorie margarine | 60 mL |

Crush the crab meat; blend with the margarine. Refrigerate overnight.

Exchange, ¼ c. (60 mL): 12 fat
Calories, ¼ c. (60 mL): 230
Carbohydrates: negligible

Garlic

¼ t.	garlic	2 mL
dash	salt	dash
¼ c.	low-calorie margarine	60 mL

Blend ingredients together.

Exchange, ¼ c. (60 mL): 12 fat
Calories, ¼ c. (60 mL): 200
Carbohydrates, ¼ c. (60 mL): negligible

Lemon

1 t.	lemon juice	5 mL
dash	salt	dash
¼ t.	parsley, chopped	1 mL
¼ c.	low-calorie margarine	60 mL

Blend ingredients together.

Exchange, ¼ c. (60 mL): 12 fat
Calories, ¼ c. (60 mL): 200
Carbohydrates, ¼ c. (60 mL): negligible

Caviar

Caviar may sound extravagant, but a little goes a long way. There are some very good domestic red or black caviars. I have even seen and bought orange, brown, light yellow caviars, and lump roe that were really very nice.

To serve caviar, bed the jars or small bowls in crushed or cracked ice. (I often use small glass custard cups or sauce bowls.) If the ice has to last a long time, I use more ice, as follows: half-fill a large serving bowl with water and place it in the refrigerator freezer. When it is frozen, spread crushed or cracked ice on top of the frozen layer; then wedge the small bowls of caviar into the crushed ice. Serve caviar with a variety of breads, crackers, wafers, or chips.

Exchange, 3½ oz. (100 g) or 20 servings: ¼ lean meat per serving
Calories, 3½ oz. (100 g) or 20 servings: 13 per serving
Carbohydrates, 3½ oz. (100 g) or 20 servings: negligible

Caviar Mounds

¼ c.	cream cheese	60 mL
5 t.	caviar	25 mL
20	crispy round crackers	20

Using a teaspoon as a mould, form the cream cheese into 20 mounds. Spread caviar on the curved side of each mound. Arrange on a plate and refrigerate until serving time. Place each mound on a cracker before serving.

Yield: 20 canapés
Exchange, 1 canapé: ⅕ fat
Calories, 1 canapé: 9
Carbohydrates, 1 canapé: negligible

Caviar-Stuffed Mushrooms

20	medium snow-white mushrooms	20
5 t.	black or red caviar	25 mL

Clean the mushrooms and remove the stems; finely chop the stems. Fill the mushroom cavities with the chopped stems. Top each mushroom with ¼ t. (1 mL) of the caviar. Chill until serving time.

Yield: 20 canapés
Exchange, 1 canapé: negligible
Calories, 1 canapé: 5
Carbohydrates, 1 canapé: negligible

Norwegian Pickled Herring

An adaption of a traditional Nordic family recipe.

8 (6 oz. each)	salt herring fillets	8 (240 g each)
1 qt.	water	1 L
½ c.	granulated sugar replacement	125 mL
¼ c.	granulated fructose	60 mL
1 c.	distilled white vinegar	250 mL
5	medium carrots, pared	5
2	medium white onions, finely chopped	2

Cut each herring crosswise into 4 pieces. Place the herring in a large glass or earthenware bowl or jar. Add enough cold water to cover. Soak for 6 hours, changing the water occasionally. Drain thoroughly. In a large noncorrosive saucepan, heat the water, sugar replacement, and fructose to the boiling point. Reduce heat and simmer for 10 minutes. Add the vinegar and reheat; simmer for 5 minutes longer. Cool to room temperature. Cut carrots into ¼-inch (6-mm) slices. Cook until just tender. Rinse under cool water. Combine the herring, carrots, and onions in a glass or earthenware bowl or jar. Cover with the sweetened mixture and stir to mix. Refrigerate, covered, until the herring are well flavored and their texture is moist and tender, about 3 days; stir occasionally. To serve, lift the herring and vegetables with a slotted spoon and arrange on a platter.

Yield: 24 servings
Exchange, 1 serving: 1 lean meat
Calories, 1 serving: 64
Carbohydrates, 1 serving: 1 g

Cottage Cheese and Shrimp Dip

½ lb.	fresh shrimp	240 g
1 c.	low-fat (1%) cottage cheese	250 mL
3 T.	cocktail sauce (from a jar)	45 mL
½ t.	onion juice	2 mL
½ t.	lemon juice	2 mL
½ t.	Worcestershire sauce	2 mL
3 T.	skim milk	45 mL
	salt (optional)	

Cook, shell, and finely chop the shrimp. To make the dip, combine all remaining ingredients and beat to a creamy consistency. Add salt, if desired. Chill thoroughly.

Yield: 2 c. (500 mL) or 32 servings

Exchange, 1 serving: $1/6$ *fat*
Calories, 1 serving: 12
Carbohydrates, 1 serving: negligible

Lobster Cocktail

A beautiful start to any meal (unless it's a fish dinner).

½ c.	white onion, finely chopped	125 mL
1 T.	fresh parsley, finely chopped	15 mL
2 t.	capers	10 mL
3 t.	sweet relish	15 mL
2	anchovy fillets	2
1	egg, hard-cooked and finely chopped	1
2¼ lbs.	lobster meat, cooked	1 kg
½ c.	low-calorie mayonnaise	125 mL
2 T.	tomato paste	30 mL
2 t.	Worcestershire sauce	10 mL
3 T.	orange juice concentrate	45 mL
1 t.	lemon juice, freshly squeezed	5 mL
2 t.	Dijon-style mustard	10 mL
2 t.	horseradish	10 mL
2 T.	dry sherry	30 mL
2 T.	cognac	30 mL
1 head	lettuce, cleaned and finely cut	1 head
	salt and fresh lemon juice	
	fresh parsley and/or lemon wedges for garnish (optional)	

Combine onion, parsley, capers, relish, anchovy fillets, and egg in a mixing bowl; stir to blend. Shred enough lobster meat to make 1 c. (250 mL). Add the lobster to the mixture with all remaining ingredients except the lettuce. Fold to blend. Season with salt and pepper, if needed. Refrigerate the mix and remaining lobster meat until thoroughly chilled. Season the lettuce with salt and lemon juice. Just before serving, divide lettuce equally among 12 margarita glasses. Place remaining lobster pieces on the lettuce bed. Top with the sauce. Garnish with a fresh sprig of parsley and/or lemon wedge, if desired.

Yield: 12 servings
Exchange, 1 serving: 1 medium-fat milk
              ⅓ bread
              ⅓ vegetable
Calories, 1 serving: 105
Carbohydrates, 1 serving: 3 g

Pickled Mushrooms

¼ lb.	snow-white mushrooms	120 g
½ c.	red wine vinegar	125 mL
¼ c.	water	60 mL
1	small white onion, cut in small wedges	1
2 t.	fresh parsley, chopped	10 mL
2 t.	granulated fructose	10 mL
1 t.	salt	5 mL
1 t.	Dijon-style mustard	5 mL

Clean the mushrooms and remove the stems; set aside. In a saucepan, combine the vinegar, water, onion, parsley, fructose, salt, and mustard. Bring to the boil and add the mushroom crowns. Simmer for 10 to 12 minutes or until the crowns are al dente. Remove from heat and chill several hours; stir occasionally. Serve cold.

Yield: 8 servings
Exchange, 1 serving: ½ vegetable
Calories, 1 serving: 12
Carbohydrates, 1 serving: 2 g

Magnificent Crab

Delicious.

2 T.	Diet Fleischmann's margarine	30 mL
1	small onion, finely chopped	1
2 t.	green bell pepper, finely chopped	10 mL
1 t.	red bell pepper, finely chopped	5 mL
½ c.	skim evaporated milk	125 mL
½ c.	skim milk	125 mL
2 T.	all-purpose flour	30 mL
2 T.	dry sherry	30 mL
½ c.	low-calorie mayonnaise	125 mL
1 T.	lemon juice, freshly squeezed	15 mL
½ t.	white pepper	2 mL
	salt to taste	
1 lb.	lump crab meat	500 g
	paprika for sprinkling	

Melt the margarine in a nonstick skillet. Sauté onions until lightly browned; reduce the heat. Add the chopped peppers and evaporated milk. Combine the flour and milk in a shaker bottle and blend thoroughly. Stir into the skillet and cook until thick and smooth; remove from the heat. Stir in the sherry, mayonnaise, lemon juice, pepper, and salt; blend well. Fold in the crab meat carefully to avoid breaking the chunks. Spoon into 8 ramekins and sprinkle with paprika. Bake at 450 °F (230 °C) until mixture is bubbling and lightly browned. Serve immediately.

Yield: 8 servings
Exchange, 1 serving: 1 lean meat
Calories, 1 serving: 83
Carbohydrates, 1 serving: 4 g

Turkey and Pork Pâté

Although this is not a true pâté because I have eliminated many of the calories by not baking it in a fat base, I think you will enjoy its flavor and texture.

4 oz.	*turkey liver, heart, and gizzard*	*120 g*
5 oz.	*pork, cut in cubes*	*150 g*
2	*garlic cloves*	*2*
⅓ c.	*onion, chopped*	*90 mL*
¼ t.	*nutmeg, freshly ground*	*1 mL*
⅛ t.	*ground ginger*	*½ mL*
½ c.	*water*	*125 mL.*

Cut the fat and membrane from the gizzard; slice the liver and heart into small pieces. In a food processor fitted with the steel blade, blend on high speed the turkey pieces, pork cubes, garlic, onion, nutmeg, ginger, and 2 T. (30 mL) of the water. Add the remaining water, a tablespoonful at a time, through the feed tube until the mixture is puréed. Turn into a 3-in. (7.6-cm) mini-loaf pan or 2-c. (500-mL) baking dish. Set the pan into a larger pan and half fill the outer pan with water. Bake at 375 °F (190 °C) for an hour or until a pick inserted in the middle comes out clean. Remove the pan from the water bath. Pour off the excess grease and turn out onto a cooling rack; place a paper towel or plate under the rack to catch dripping grease. Cool to room temperature. With a sharp knife, cut into 15 slices; cut each slice in half. If desired, serve with crackers or thin rye bread.

Yield: 30 servings
Exchange, 1 serving (without bread): ⅓ lean meat
Calories, 1 serving (without bread): 15
Carbohydrates, 1 serving (without bread): negligible

Fried Shrimp

2 T.	all-purpose flour	30 mL
1 T.	cornstarch	15 mL
1 t.	soy sauce	5 mL
1 T.	red wine vinegar	15 mL
2	eggs, well beaten	2
½ t.	salt	2 mL
¼ t.	freshly ground black pepper	1 mL
	oil for frying	
20	large fresh shrimp	20

Combine the flour, cornstarch, soy sauce, vinegar, eggs, salt, and pepper in a deep bowl; beat well to blend the batter. Heat oil to 375 °F (190 °C) in a saucepan or deep fryer. Dip shrimp into the batter and shake off the excess; then gently drop into the hot oil. Cook 15 to 20 seconds or until browned. Remove with a slotted spoon and drain well. Keep warm or serve immediately.

Yield: 20 servings
Exchange, 1 serving: 1 lean meat
Calories, 1 serving: 63
Carbohydrates, 1 serving: 4 g

Shrimp Cocktail

1 lb.	large shrimp tails in their shells	500 g
1	bay leaf	1
1	small white onion, sliced	1
¼ t.	celery seeds, crushed	1 mL

To shell the shrimp: hold the tail end in the left hand; slip your free thumb under the shell; then holding firmly to the tail, pull out the shrimp. With a sharp knife, cut along the outside curve of shrimp and lift out black vein. Wash shrimp under water. Drop shrimp and remaining ingredients into boiling salted water. Simmer, covered, for 2 to 4 minutes or until pink. Drain and chill thoroughly. Place chilled shrimp on a bed of ice or lettuce leaves. Serve cold.

Yield: 5 servings
Exchange, 1 serving: 1 lean meat
Calories, 1 serving: 57
Carbohydrates, 1 serving: 1 g

Kabobs of Beef

1 lb.	lean ground round beef	500 g
⅓ c.	onion, finely chopped	90 mL
¼ c.	fresh bread crumbs	60 mL
3 T.	coriander leaves, finely chopped	45 mL
2 t.	fresh ginger, grated	10 mL
1 t.	lemon juice, freshly squeezed	5 mL
2	hot chilies, cleaned and finely chopped	2
2	eggs	2
2	garlic cloves, minced	2
	salt and freshly ground pepper to taste	

Combine all ingredients in a large mixing bowl. With your hands, blend thoroughly. Form into a large ball. Wrap tightly in plastic wrap and refrigerate overnight. Using a tablespoon form into 45 small balls. Sauté in a nonstick skillet over low heat until brown. Roll balls or shake the skillet often to avoid sticking. Serve immediately or keep warm. (If the kabobs are planned for a cocktail party, serve them in a chafing dish with ½ c. (125 mL) hot beef stock on the bottom.) ·

Yield: 45 kabobs
Exchange, 2 kabobs: ½ lean meat
Calories, 2 kabobs: 30
Carbohydrates, 2 kabobs: negligible

Salads

Ethnic, regional, and individual tastes dictate when a salad should be served. Salads can be served before, during, or following a main course. In many countries, the salad is enjoyed as an hors d'oeuvre. Salads, both hot and cold, can vary from a simple lettuce arrangement to a main dish, such as chef salad. Whatever their ingredients and whenever they are served, salads should be moist and planned as a complement to the meal.

If you are serving an elaborate or heavy entrée, keep your salad light and colorful. An assortment of lettuces with a garnish is a very suitable salad for most meat and seafood dinners. Decorating green salads with vegetable garnishes will add the interest and color you need. Some of the simplest garnishes, such as the following examples, are also the easiest to make.

Radish rose: Trim off all or most of the stem and cut off the root end of a radish. With a thin, sharp knife, cut the outside red layer almost down to the stem end in 5 or more sections. Chill thoroughly in ice water. The layers will stand out like petals of a flower.

Carrot curls: Clean and slice a large carrot in half lengthwise. Using a vegetable peeler, slice down the cut side of the carrot. Roll the thin carrot strips into curls; secure each curl with a toothpick. Chill in ice water.

Turnip lily: Clean and cut a turnip into thin slices. Form each slice into a cone or cornucopia. Place a thin slice of carrot or green bean into the opening. Secure the base by fastening it with a toothpick. Dip the flower into warm clear gelatin and place on a rack. Refrigerate until set.

Vegetable fan: Cut uncooked carrots, celery, turnips, squash, or green or red peppers into thin julienne strips. Chill in ice water. Place the strips inside a ring of onions or green or red pepper and arrange in a fan shape on a bed of lettuce.

Bouillon aux Legumes

2 env.	unflavored gelatin	2 env.
1 c.	cold water	250 mL
1 c.	rich chicken bouillon or stock	250 mL
1½ t.	white vinegar	7 mL
½ t.	salt	2 mL
¼ t.	paprika	1 mL
1 c.	red cabbage, finely shredded	250 mL
¼ c.	celery, paper-thinly sliced	60 mL
¼ c.	green pepper, finely chopped	60 mL
2 c.	spinach, finely chopped	500 mL

Soften gelatin in the cold water in a saucepan. Add the chicken stock, vinegar, salt, and paprika. Bring to the boil to dissolve gelatin. Cool to room temperature until gelatin sets slightly. Fold in the vegetables. Pour into individual moulds that have been coated with a shortening or spray. Chill until firm. Unmould onto small plates. Encircle with chopped spinach.

Yield: 4 servings
Exchange, 1 serving: 1 vegetable
Calories, 1 serving: 20
Carbohydrates, 1 serving: 5 g

Red Onion and Orange Salad

A tasty salad with a slightly Spanish flavor.

2	Boston lettuce heads	2
1	small red onion, cut in rings	1
4	oranges, peeled and sliced in rings	4
1 recipe	Cilantro Dressing	1 recipe

Remove the stems from lettuce and wash thoroughly; drain. Carefully separate the leaves to keep them whole. Place leaves in plastic bags or refrigerator container. Chill for at least 2 hours. Line 6 chilled salad plates with lettuce. Arrange onion rings alternately with orange rings on the lettuce base. Spoon dressing over the salad.

Yield: 6 servings
Exchange, 1 serving: 1 fruit
*   1 vegetable*
Calories, 1 serving: 61
Carbohydrates, 1 serving: 14 g

Oriental Platter

A lovely color addition for your table. Remember, much of gourmet cooking is the way it is presented.

2 t.	salt	10 mL
2 c.	cucumbers, very thinly cut	500 mL
2 c.	carrots, finely shredded	500 mL
¼ t.	salt	1 mL
2 env.	Equal low-calorie sweetener	2 env.
½ c.	white vinegar	125 mL
1 c.	radishes, very thinly cut	250 mL
8	lettuce leaves	8

Sprinkle salt over the cucumbers. Refrigerate for at least 2 hours. Drain thoroughly. Place in paper or kitchen towel; press to remove excess moisture. Combine the salt, sweetener, and vinegar in a bowl. Pour over the carrots. Refrigerate for at least an hour. Drain the marinade from the carrots into a serving bowl to serve as a dressing. Place a lettuce leaf on each plate or salad platter. Heap cucumbers in the middle; circle half of the platter with carrots, the other half with radishes. Serve immediately or cover and refrigerate.

Yield: 8 servings
Exchange, 1 serving: ¾ vegetable
Calories, 1 serving: 15
Carbohydrates, 1 serving: 4 g

Squid and Bay Scallop Salad

1 lb.	squid	500 g
½ lb.	bay scallops	250 g
½ c.	water	125 mL
¼ c.	red wine vinegar	60 mL
8	peppercorns	8
1	bay leaf	1
2 t.	salt	10 mL
½ c.	celery, sliced	125 mL
¼ c.	green pepper, chopped	60 mL
¼ c.	endive, chopped	60 mL
2 T.	light olive oil	30 mL
2	cloves garlic, minced	2
3 T.	lemon juice, freshly squeezed	45 mL

Clean the squid* and cut bodies and tentacles into rings. Combine squid, scallops, water, half of the vinegar, peppercorns, bay leaf, and salt in a saucepan. Bring to the boil, cover, and boil for 2 to 3 minutes; drain thoroughly. Remove the squid and scallops and discard the peppercorns and bay leaf. Combine the squid, scallops, celery, green pepper, endive, oil, garlic, lemon juice and remaining vinegar in a bowl; toss to coat. Cover and cool to room temperature.

*To clean squid: Rinse in cold water, place fingers at eyes, pinch and pull off the head (most of the interior will come out with the head). Cut off and discard the eyes and cartilaginous ball between them. Clean out any remaining interior and the slender translucent support shaped like a pen and discard. Under cold water rinse and rub the squid with your fingers to loosen the skin and pull it off. Rinse thoroughly. Prepare as directed in the recipe.

Yield: 8 servings
Exchange, 1 serving: 1 lean meat
½ vegetable
Calories, 1 serving: 68
Carbohydrates, 1 serving: 2 g

Hot Red Cabbage

This could be used as either a salad or vegetable. It is particularly good with pork.

2 c.	water	500 mL
2 T.	vegetable oil	30 mL
1 qt.	red cabbage, shredded	1 L
2	medium apples, chopped coarsely	2
⅔ c.	cider vinegar	180 mL
½ t.	salt	2 mL
2 env.	Equal low-calorie sweetener	2 env.

Combine water, oil, cabbage, apples, vinegar, and salt in a saucepan. Bring to the boil. Reduce heat and simmer until apple is tender. Drain thoroughly. Sprinkle with the sweetener; toss to mix. Serve immediately.

Yield: 8 servings
Exchange, 1 serving: 1 fat
1 vegetable
Calories, 1 serving: 68
Carbohydrates, 1 serving: 9 g

Salad Basics

I like to keep a combination of these salad greens on hand at all times. Wash and break about 6 c. (1.5 L) into bite-size pieces. Store them in an airtight refrigerator bowl. It is an easy and simple way to come up with a salad for every meal.

iceberg lettuce	endive
Bibb lettuce	watercress
romaine	celery cabbage
leaf lettuce	celery leaves
escarole	spinach leaves
Boston lettuce	

Exchange, 1 c. (250 mL): negligible
Calories, 1 c. (250 mL): 5
Carbohydrates, 1 c. (250 mL): 2 g

Green Salad with Oregano

6 c.	Salad Basics	1.5 L
half	white onion, sliced in rings	half
2 t.	fresh or ½ t. (2 mL) dried oregano	10 mL
2 T.	light olive oil	30 mL
2 T.	red wine vinegar	30 mL
1 T.	Dijon-style mustard	15 mL
1 T.	green onion, finely chopped	15 mL
½ t.	salt	2 mL
¼ t.	black pepper, freshly ground	1 mL

Place the mixed salad basics and onion rings in a salad bowl. Sprinkle with oregano. Combine the oil, vinegar, mustard, green onion, salt, and pepper in a mixing bowl. With an electric mixer, beat on HIGH for 5 minutes. Pour the dressing over the salad and toss well.

Yield: 6 servings
Exchange, 1 serving: 1 fat
Calories, 1 serving: 40
Carbohydrates, 1 serving: 2 g

Salad with Corn and Artichokes

1 c.	fresh white corn kernels	250 mL
14-oz. jar	marinated artichoke hearts	420-g jar

½	sweet red pepper, cut in thin strips	125 mL
3 T.	white wine vinegar	45 mL
1	clove garlic, minced	1
½ t.	dried oregano, crumbled	2 mL
3 c.	Salad Basics	750 mL

Combine corn, artichoke hearts with the marinade (cut artichokes, if large), pepper strips, vinegar, garlic, and oregano in a refrigerator bowl with a tight lid; shake to coat the vegetables. Refrigerate for at least 2 hours. Place salad basics in a chilled salad bowl. Just before serving, pour marinated vegetables over the top.

Yield: 8 servings
Exchange, 1 serving: 1 vegetable
Calories, 1 serving: 30
Carbohydrates, 1 serving: 7 g

Royal Fruit

1 c.	mandarin orange sections	250 mL
1 c.	grapefruit sections	250 mL
¼ lb.	seedless green grapes	125 g
¼ lb.	seedless red grapes	125 g
½ c.	white wine	125 mL
½ t.	orange peel slivers	2 mL
1 in.	vanilla bean	2.5 cm
2 c.	Salad Basics	500 mL
2	kiwis, sliced	2

Combine the orange and grapefruit sections and the grapes in a medium-sized bowl. Combine the wine, orange peel, and vanilla bean in a small saucepan and heat just to the boiling point. Pour over the fruits in the bowl; cover and cool to room temperature. Place a ⅓-c. (90-mL) bed of salad basics on each of 6 chilled salad plates. Remove the vanilla bean from the fruit. Using a slotted spoon, divide the fruit equally among the plates. Garnish with kiwi slices.

Yield: 6 servings
Exchange, 1 serving: 1 fruit
Calories, 1 serving: 41
Carbohydrates, 1 serving: 10 g

Choice Fruit Salad

2 T.	lemon juice	30 mL
½ c.	water	125 mL
4	medium Delicious apples	4
2	bananas	2
¼ t.	unflavored gelatin	1 mL
2 pkg.	Equal low-calorie sweetener	2 pkg.
10	strawberries	10

Combine the lemon juice and a small amount of water in a glass bowl. Peel and core the apples. Slice directly into lemon water. Peel and slice the bananas into the lemon water. Fold slightly to coat the fruits and rest for 5 minutes. Meanwhile, combine the ½ c. (125 mL) water and gelatin in a small saucepan. Bring to the boil, reduce heat, and simmer for 2 minutes. Remove from heat and cool. When cool enough to place your hand on the bottom of the pan, stir in the sweetener. Drain apple and banana slices thoroughly. Wash and slice strawberries and stir into the apple-banana mixture. Pour the sweetened gelatin over the top and fold gently to coat the mixture. Refrigerate until chilled.

Yield: 7 servings
Exchange, 1 serving: 2 fruit
Calories, 1 serving: 80
Carbohydrates, 1 serving: 20 g

Summer Shrimp Salad

8 oz.	rotini pasta	226 g
⅓ c.	white onions, chopped	90 mL
1 c.	celery, thinly sliced	250 mL
1 c.	frozen green peas	250 mL
6-oz. bag	small frozen shrimp	170-g bag
1 c.	low-calorie salad dressing	250 mL
3 T.	skim evaporated milk	45 mL

Cook pasta as directed on the package; drain thoroughly. While hot, add the remaining ingredients; fold to blend. Place in a glass serving dish; cover tightly. Refrigerate until chilled or overnight.

Yield: 8 servings
Exchange, 1 serving: 2 bread
*   1 fat*
Calories, 1 serving: 182
Carbohydrates, 1 serving: 28 g

Peach and Shrimp Salad

4	fresh peaches	4
1 T.	lemon juice	15 mL
1½ c.	low-calorie cottage cheese	375 mL
6-oz. bag	Brilliant cooked shrimp, thawed and drained	170-g bag
½ t.	salt	2 mL
1 env.	aspartame sweetener	1 env.

Peel and cut peaches in half; remove the pits. Sprinkle each half with lemon juice. With the back of the hand or the bottom of a plate, flatten peaches slightly. Place in champagne glasses. Combine the remaining ingredients and fold to blend. Pile over the peaches. Garnish with mint leaves.

Yield: 8 servings
Exchange, 1 serving: ¾ lean meat
½ fruit
Calories, 1 serving: 62
Carbohydrates, 1 serving: 6 g

Grapefuit and Apple Salad

2 env.	unflavored gelatin	2 env.
1 c.	unsweetened grapefruit juice	250 mL
¼ c.	lemon juice, freshly squeezed	60 mL
2 c.	water	500 mL
⅛ t.	salt	½ mL
3 env.	Equal low-calorie sweetener	3 env.
2 c.	grapefruit sections, with seeds and membranes removed	500 mL
2	medium red Delicious apples, sliced with peels on watercress for garnish	2

Soften gelatin in the grapefruit juice in a saucepan. Add the lemon juice, water, and salt. Bring to the boil, reduce heat, and stir to dissolve the gelatin. Remove from heat and cool until thickened. Add the sweetener and stir to dissolve. Fold in the fruits. Rinse a 5-c. (1.25-L) mould with cold water. Pour in the fruit mixture and chill until firm. Turn out on a chilled serving platter. Garnish with a circle of watercress.

Yield: 10 servings
Exchange, 1 serving: 1 fruit
Calories, 1 serving: 36
Carbohydrates, 1 serving: 8 g

Cherry Tomato and Mushroom Salad

¾ lb.	small snow mushroom caps	365 g
3 T.	light olive oil	45 mL
1 T.	dry white wine	15 mL
2 T.	lemon juice, freshly squeezed	30 mL
½ t.	salt	2 mL
¼ t.	black pepper, freshly ground	1 mL
20	cherry tomatoes, sliced in half	20
3 T.	fresh chive, chopped	45 mL
10	curly leafed lettuce leaves, cleaned	10

Clean and wipe the mushrooms with a damp towel or a mushroom brush (if you cannot get small caps, cut large mushrooms in halves or quarters). Place mushrooms in a bowl. Blend the oil, wine, lemon juice, salt, and pepper in a bowl and pour over the mushrooms. Cover and marinate for at least 3 hours or overnight. Just before serving, add tomato halves to the mushroom mixture; toss lightly to coat tomatoes with the dressing. Chill 5 salad plates; place 2 lettuce leaves on each. Divide mushroom mixture evenly among the plates. Serve immediately.

Yield: 5 servings
Exchange, 1 serving: 1 vegetable
1 fat
Calories, 1 serving: 76
Carbohydrates, 1 serving: 7 g

Cilantro Dressing

A green dressing with a light Spanish flavor.

⅓ c.	orange juice	90 mL
2 T.	red wine vinegar	30 mL
1 t.	Dijon-style mustard	5 mL
1 T.	cilantro (coriander) leaves, chopped	15 mL

Combine all ingredients in a blender and blend for at least 5 minutes. Refrigerate until ready to use. Shake just before using.

Yield: ⅓ c. (90 mL) or 3 servings
Exchange, 1 serving: ⅓ fruit
Calories, 1 serving: 12
Carbohydrates, 1 serving: 3 g

Burgundy Vinaigrette

½ c.	cold water	125 mL
1 t.	cornstarch	5 mL
¼ c.	Burgundy	60 mL
1½ t.	white vinegar	7 mL
¼ t.	smooth-leaf parsley	1 mL
⅛ t.	Italian oregano	½ mL
dash	garlic powder	dash
1 env.	Equal low-calorie sweetener	1 env.

Combine the water and cornstarch in a small saucepan and stir to blend. Cook over medium heat until clear. Add the wine, vinegar, parsley, oregano, and garlic powder and cook for 3 minutes; remove from heat. When you can place your hand on the bottom of the saucepan, stir in the sweetener. Refrigerate until chilled.

Yield: ⅔ c. (180 mL) or 6 servings
Exchange, 1 serving: negligible
Calories, 1 serving: negligible
Carbohydrates, 1 serving: ⅔ g

French Dressing

½ c.	cold water	125 mL
1 T.	cornstarch	15 mL
½ c.	vegetable oil	125 mL
¼ c.	white vinegar	60 mL
½ t.	salt	2 mL
¼ t.	white pepper	1 mL
⅛ t.	cayenne pepper	½ mL
2 T.	parsley, finely snipped	30 mL

Combine water and cornstarch in a small saucepan. Cook and stir over medium heat until clear and thickened; cool slightly. Combine the cornstarch liquid and remaining ingredients in a blender. Beat to thoroughly blend. Chill thoroughly.

Yield: 1¼ c. (310 mL) or 20 servings
Exchange, 1 serving: 1 fat
Calories, 1 serving: 50
Carbohydrates, 1 serving: negligible

Soups and Stews

There is no limit to the kinds and numbers of soups but generally they are classified into three groups:

1. Thin, clear soups such as broths or stocks, bouillons and consommés. A bouillon is a broth made by simmering vegetables and fish, poultry, or meat to extract the flavors; consommé is a clear bouillon.

2. Thin, delicately light soups, such as light cream soups and bisques.

3. Heavy, thick soups, such as meat or vegetable soups, including minestrone, chowders, or thick cream soups. Like stews, these soups can be served as the main course.

Jelled or chilled soup can fall into any of these categories.

Stews are any dishes prepared in water by a slow cooking with simmering heat. Today, many of us consider a stew as having a meat and one or more vegetables. We also like to thicken the broth for a gravy to the dish.

Chicken Stock

4¼ lbs.	chicken parts, wings, backs, and necks	2 kg
4 qts.	water	4 L
1	large onion, quartered	1
1	large carrot, cut in chucks	1
1 c.	celery, cut in chucks	250 mL
1	parsley sprig, chopped	1
½ t.	poultry seasoning	2 mL

Combine all ingredients in a soup pot and heat to the boiling point. Reduce the heat and simmer for 4 hours; add extra water, if needed. Strain stock through a sieve and discard meat and vegetable solids; cool.

Refrigerate, allowing the fat to conqeal on the surface. Remove and discard the fat. Use the stock as directed in the recipes.

Yield: 4 qts. (4 L)
Exchange: negligible
Calories: negligible
Carbohydrates: negligible

Beef Stock

4½ lbs.	beef neck bones	2 kg
2	large yellow onions	2
3	carrots	3
3	celery ribs with leaves	3
2	garlic cloves	2
3	fresh parsley sprigs	3
3	bay leaves	3
4 qts.	water	4 L

Clean the onions, carrots, and celery and cut into chucks. Combine the beef bones, onions, carrots, and celery in a large roasting pan. Roast at 400 °F (200 °C) for about 50 minutes or until bones are a deep brown color. Turn the bones and vegetables into a large soup pot. Rinse out the roaster with some of the water, scraping the bottom and sides of pan with a wooden spoon to remove any browned particles; add to soup pot. Add the remaining ingredients and water. Cook over medium heat to the boiling point; reduce heat and simmer for about 5 hours, adding extra water, if needed. Strain stock through a sieve, and discard the meat and vegetable solids; cool. Refrigerate, allowing the fat to congeal on the surface; remove and discard the fat. Use the stock as directed in the recipes.

Yield: 4 qts. (4 L)
Exchange: negligible
Calories: negligible
Carbohydrates: negligible

Fish Stock

2½ lbs.	fresh lean fish (flounder, sole, or whiting)	1 kg
1	onion, thinly sliced	1
2 t.	lemon juice, freshly squeezed	10 mL
1 c.	dry white wine	250 mL

1½ c.	water	375 mL
¼ t.	salt	1 mL
	freshly ground black pepper	

Combine all the ingredients except salt and pepper in a soup pot or Dutch oven. Cover and simmer for 30 to 40 minutes. Strain and season to taste with salt and pepper. (The fish meat may be used for other recipes. Remove fish meat from the bones and discard bones, heads, and tails.)

Yield: 2 c. (500 mL)
Exchange: negligible
Calories: negligible
Carbohydrates: negligible

Champignon Soup

1 each	chicken neck, liver, and gizzard	1 each
2½ c.	water	750 mL
5	green onions with 3 in. (7.5 cm) of green*	5
⅓ c.	dried black mushrooms, soaked and sliced	90 mL
2 t.	cornstarch	10 mL
2 T.	skim evaporated milk	30 mL
1 t.	salt	5 mL
	black pepper, freshly ground	

Combine chicken parts and water in a medium saucepan. Bring to the boil, reduce heat, and simmer for 30 to 40 minutes; strain. Set meat aside to cool. Chill the stock and remove and discard fat. Cut onions into ½ in. (13-mm) slices. Add the onions and mushrooms to the stock. Simmer for 15 minutes. Blend the cornstarch with the milk and slowly stir into the soup. Remove meat from neck bone, discarding the skin and bone. Chop liver and gizzard; discard tendon from the gizzard. Add meat, liver, gizzard, and salt to the soup. Cook and stir over low heat until broth is clear (the broth will thicken only slightly). Season the soup with pepper to taste.

*If unavailable, use leeks.

Yield: 2 soup-bowl servings or 4 soup-cup servings
Exchange, 1 soup-bowl serving: ½ vegetable
Calories, 1 soup-bowl serving: 17
Carbohydrates, 1 soup-bowl serving: 4 g
Exchange, 1 soup-cup serving: ¼ vegetable
Calories, 1 soup-cup serving: 8
Carbohydrates, 1 soup-cup serving: 2 g

Chive and Mushroom Bisque

This bisque is unique in that it uses rice as both the base of the soup and the thickening agent.

1½ c.	cooked rice	375 mL
1 qt.	water	1 L
¼ c.	chive, chopped	60 mL
1½ c.	celery, finely chopped	375 mL
¼ lb.	mushrooms, finely chopped	120 g
1 t.	salt	5 mL
	freshly ground pepper to taste	
5 T.	Dannon plain low-fat yogurt	75 mL

Combine cooked rice and 1 c. (250 mL) of the water in a blender. Blend until completely puréed. Pour into a nonstick saucepan. Add the remaining water, chive, celery, mushrooms, salt, and pepper. Cook and stir over medium heat until vegetables are cooked and soup is thickened. Serve immediately. If desired, top each serving with 1 T. (15 mL) yogurt.

Yield: 5 servings
Exchange, 1 serving: 1 bread
Calories, 1 serving: 80
Carbohydrates, 1 serving: 16 g

Baked Onion Soup

2 T.	low-calorie margarine	30 mL
4	large white onions, thinly sliced	4
1 qt.	Beef Stock (homemade) or canned beef broth	1 L
4	French Bread slices (homemade), toasted	4
2	Gruyère cheese slices, cut in strips	2

Melt margarine in a skillet and sauté the onions until brown. Add the stock and simmer for 5 minutes. Place toast in 4 ovenproof soup bowls. Ladle hot soup over the toast. Top with cheese strips. Bake at 350 °F (175 °C) for 25 to 30 minutes.

Yield: 4 servings
Exchange, 1 serving: 1 bread
1 high-fat meat
1 vegetable
Calories, 1 serving: 195
Carbohydrates, 1 serving: 23 g

Bouillabaisse

One of the world's great soups—a highly seasoned fish stew.

2¼ lbs.	assorted fish (such as whiting, red snapper, sole, flounder, and a small amount of eel)	1 kg
1 lb.	lobster	500 g
1 lb.	shrimp	450 g
24	mussels	24
12	clams	12
¼ c.	olive oil	60 mL
3	leek bulbs, chopped	3
2	onions, chopped	2
3	garlic cloves, sliced	3
3	large tomatoes, peeled, seeded, and chopped	3
1	bouquet garni (bay leaf, thyme, and parsley)	1
dash	saffron	dash
	salt, black pepper, and cayenne pepper	

Clean and cut the fish and lobster into serving pieces. Clean the shrimp and scrub the mussels and clams. Heat the oil in a large soup pot or Dutch oven. Sauté leeks, onions, garlic, and tomatoes for 2 minutes. Add the bouquet garni, saffron, and heavy fish such as eel, haddock, or halibut; cover and boil for 7 minutes. Add remaining fish, lobster, and enough boiling water to cover the fish. Cover and boil for 10 minutes. Add the mussels and clams, cover, and boil until they open (discard any that do not open). Add the shrimp, reduce heat, and simmer for 15 minutes; remove bouquet garni. Ladle soup into heated serving bowls. (Toast, French bread, or croutons may be served with the soup, if desired.)

Yield: 20 servings
Exchange, 1 serving: 1½ lean meat
½ vegetable
Calories, 1 serving: 101
Carbohydrates, 1 serving: 2 g

Turtle Soup with Sherry

3 T.	unsalted butter	45 mL
1 lb.	turtle meat, cut in ½-in. (1.25-cm) cubes	500 g
1	large onion, chopped	1
½ c.	celery with leaves, chopped	125 mL
⅓ c.	carrot, finely chopped	90 mL
1	garlic clove, minced	1

2 c.	tomato sauce	500 mL
1	lemon	1
1	bay leaf	1
2	parsley sprigs, snipped	2
½ c.	dry sherry	125 mL
1 qt.	Beef Stock	1 L

Melt butter in a large soup pot or Dutch oven. Sauté turtle until golden brown. Add the onion, celery, carrot, garlic, and tomato sauce. Cook and stir until onions are tender. Squeeze the juice from the lemon and add to the pot. Finely grate the lemon peel and add to the pot with remaining ingredients. Simmer gently for 1½ to 2 hours. Serve in heated soup bowls.

Yield: 8 servings
Exchange, 1 serving: 1½ lean meat
2 vegetable
Calories, 1 serving: 132
Carbohydrates, 1 serving: 8

Tomato and Crab Bisque

1 T.	butter	15 mL
2 T.	onion, finely chopped	30 mL
2 T.	all-purpose flour	30 mL
2 c.	skim milk	500 mL
1 c.	crab meat, flaked	250 mL
1 c.	tomato juice	250 mL
	salt and freshly ground pepper to taste	

Melt butter in a nonstick saucepan. Add onion and sauté until lightly browned. Add the flour and blend. Slowly add the milk and cook until partially thickened. Stir in the crab meat and tomato juice and cook over medium heat, stirring constantly, until thickened. Season to taste. Serve immediately.

Yield: 4 soup-bowl servings or 8 soup-cup servings
Exchange, 1 soup-bowl serving: 1 lean meat
¾ bread
Calories, 1 soup-bowl serving: 109
Carbohydrates, 1 soup-bowl serving: 8 g
Exchange, 1 soup-cup serving: ½ lean meat
⅓ bread
Calories, 1 soup-cup serving: 54
Carbohydrates, 1 soup-cup serving: 4 g

Vichyssoise

4	potatoes, peeled and cubed	4
1 qt.	Chicken Stock	1 L
2 T.	unsalted butter	30 mL
1	medium onion, finely chopped	1
1 c.	skim evaporated milk	250 mL
1 T.	cornstarch	15 mL
1 c.	water	250 mL
¼ c.	fresh chive	60 mL
	salt and freshly ground pepper	

Cook the potatoes in chicken stock until soft; remove from heat. Melt butter in a nonstick skillet. Stir in the onions and sauté until tender but not brown. Add to the potato mixture. In small amounts, beat the mixture in a blender or food processor until creamy; return to the soup pot. Blend the cornstarch with water and slowly stir into the soup with the evaporated milk. Return to the heat, stir, and simmer until smooth and slightly thickened. Season to taste with salt and pepper. Chill thoroughly before serving. Garnish each soup serving with chive.

Yield: 8 soup-bowl servings or 16 soup-cup servings
Exchange, 1 soup-bowl serving: 1 bread
½ fat
Calories, 1 soup-bowl serving: 103
Carbohydrates, 1 soup-bowl serving: 13 g
Exchange, 1 soup-cup serving: ½ bread
¼ fat
Calories, 1 soup-cup serving: 51
Carbohydrates, 1 soup-cup serving: 7 g

Mussel Chowder

A great entrée on a winter night.

8-oz. can	mussels, drained	240-g can
⅛ lb.	side pork, thinly sliced	63 g
1	celery stalk, with leaves, chopped	1
½ c.	leek, chopped	125 mL
1	green pepper, peeled and chopped	1
2	medium potatoes, diced	2
2	bay leaves, crushed	2
2 c.	water	500 mL

2½ c.	skim milk	625 mL
2 T.	all-purpose flour	30 mL
	salt, freshly ground pepper, and parsley	

In a large nonstick skillet, fry the pork until crisp. Remove the pork and crumble; set aside. Add the celery and leek to the skillet and sauté over medium heat until the leek begins to brown. Add the green pepper, potatoes, bay leaves, and water. Bring to the boil, reduce heat, and simmer for 10 minutes. Combine ½ c. (125 mL) of the milk with the flour and stir until smooth; blend into the chowder. Add the remaining milk and the mussels and simmer until thoroughly warmed. Season with salt and pepper to taste. Ladle the chowder into 4 soup bowls. Garnish with the parsley and crumbled pork.

Yield: 4 servings
Exchange, 1 serving: 1⅓ bread
1 medium-fat meat
1 fat
Calories, 1 serving: 195
Carbohydrates, 1 serving: 16 g

Purée of Chestnut Soup

1 T.	unsalted butter	15 mL
1	large yellow onion, chopped	1
1 lb.	chestnuts, shelled	500 g
1 qt.	hot Chicken Stock or canned chicken broth	1 L
1	celery stalk with leaves, chopped	1
1	carrot, finely diced	1
2 T.	fresh parsley, snipped	30 mL
2 T.	Madeira	30 mL
2 T.	half-and-half (cream and milk)	30 mL

Melt the butter in a soup pot and sauté the onions until brown. Add the chestnuts and sauté for 2 minutes. Stir in the stock, celery, carrot, and parsley. Cover and simmer for 40 to 45 minutes. Pour mixture into a blender and blend at high speed until puréed. Return to the pot and reheat. Just before serving, stir in the Madeira and half-and-half.

Yield: 8 servings
Exchange, 1 serving: 1⅔ bread
Calories, 1 serving: 122
Carbohydrates, 1 serving: 25 g

Fresh Green Pea Soup

2 T.	Diet Fleischmann's margarine	30 mL
1 c.	fresh green peas	250 mL
2 T.	all-purpose flour	30 mL
1 qt.	water	1 L
	salt and freshly ground pepper	
2 T.	parsley, snipped	30 mL

Melt margarine in a large soup pot or Dutch oven. Sauté the peas for 2 minutes. Combine the flour with water and shake or stir to completely blend. Stir into peas. Season with salt and pepper. Simmer gently until peas are soft. Sprinkle with parsley before serving.

Yield: 4 servings
Exchange, 1 serving: ²/₃ bread
½ fat
Calories, 1 serving: 69
Carbohydrates, 1 serving: 9 g

Curried Rice Purée

1½ c.	Chicken Stock	375 mL
¼ c.	onion, chopped	60 mL
¼ c.	carrots, grated	60 mL
1	garlic clove, minced	1
1 T.	long-grain rice	15 mL
½ c.	half-and-half (cream and milk)	125 mL
2 t.	curry powder	10 mL
	salt and freshly ground pepper to taste	

Combine the stock, onion, carrots, garlic, and rice in a saucepan. Bring to the boil, reduce heat, cover, and simmer for 35 minutes. Remove from heat and cool slightly. Pour into a blender; blend to a purée. Stir in the half-and-half and curry powder; return mixture to the saucepan and heat just to serving temperature. Season with salt and pepper to taste. Serve immediately.

Yield: 5 servings
Exchange, 1 serving: ⅓ low-fat milk
Calories, 1 serving: 44
Carbohydrates, 1 serving: 4 g

Sherry Soup

2 c.	Chicken Stock	500 mL
¼ c.	cream sherry	60 mL
½ t.	lemon juice	2 mL
½ t.	fresh lavender leaves	2 mL
	salt and freshly ground pepper	
2	spinach leaves	2
2	fresh lemon strips	2

Heat the stock, sherry, lemon juice, and lavender leaves in a saucepan. Season with salt and pepper to taste. Ladle the soup into heated soup bowls or cups. Garnish with spinach leaves and lemon strips (if using cups, cut spinach leaves and lemon strips in half).

Yield: 2 servings
Exchange, 1 serving: ⅓ bread
1 fat
Calories, 1 serving: 70
Carbohydrates, 1 serving: 4 g

Egg-Lemon Soup

6 c.	Chicken Stock	1.5 L
½ c.	long-grain rice	125 mL
3	eggs, separated	3
3 T.	lemon juice, freshly squeezed	45 mL
	fresh parsley, snipped	

In a large saucepan, bring the stock to the boiling point. Stir in the rice, reduce heat, and simmer for 15 minutes. Meanwhile, beat the egg whites until stiff. Add egg yolks to stiffly beaten egg whites, one at a time, continually beating. Beat until mixture is light yellow. Slowly add the lemon juice. Gradually stir ⅓ c. (90 mL) hot broth into the egg mixture. Slowly pour egg mixture into the hot broth while beating with a wire whisk. Spoon into hot serving bowls or cups. Garnish with the parsley.

Yield: 6 servings
Exchange, 1 serving: 1 bread
½ lean meat
Calories, 1 serving: 95
Carbohydrates, 1 serving: 13 g

Entrées

Entrée in French means "entrance" or "entering." In culinary terms, the entrée is one of the dishes of a meal and as a rule, the principal dish. In keeping with this thought, I have prepared glorious gourmet recipes from shark to shrimp, steak to chops, venison to pheasant and chicken for you. So select, cook, and enjoy.

Crab Newburg

2 T.	low-calorie margarine	30 mL
1½ c.	flaked crab meat	375 mL
2 t.	all-purpose flour	10 mL
½ c.	skim evaporated milk	125 mL
2 T.	cream sherry	30 mL
2	egg yolks, slightly beaten	2
½ t.	salt	2 mL

Melt the margarine in a saucepan, add the crab meat and sauté over low heat for 4 minutes. Combine the milk and flour in a bowl or shaker bottle and blend well. Stir into the crab meat and continue cooking, stirring constantly, until the mixture boils. Add the sherry and egg yolks. Cook and stir a minute longer; remove from the heat. Serve warm on crisp toast or Pastry Shells, if desired.

Yield: 6 servings
Exchange, 1 serving: 1 lean meat
½ fat
⅓ bread
Calories, 1 serving: 92
Carbohydrates, 1 serving: 3 g

Marinated Crab Legs

½ c.	Teriyaki Marinade	125 mL
⅓ c.	lemon juice	90 mL
½ c.	water	125 mL
1 t.	basil	5 mL
1 lb.	cooked crab meat from the legs	500 g

Mix the marinade, lemon juice, water, and basil. Add the crab meat (if necessary, add more water to cover the crab meat). Marinate for 2 to 3 hours in the refrigerator. Serve cold.

Yield: 8 servings
Exchange, 1 serving: 1 lean meat
Calories, 1 serving: 52
Carbohydrates, 1 serving: negligible

Shrimp de Jonghe

This seafood delight developed in Chicago.

1 lb.	shrimps	500 g
2 T.	white wine	30 mL
1	garlic clove, minced	1
2 t.	unsalted butter	10 mL
¼ t.	leek, finely snipped	1 mL
¼ t.	salt	1 mL
⅛ t.	fresh tarragon leaves	½ mL
⅛ t.	parsley, finely snipped	½ mL
dash of each	freshly ground pepper and allspice, dried thyme, and grated nutmeg	dash of each
⅓ c.	bread crumbs	90 mL

Clean and rinse the shrimps. Arrange shrimps in 4 shell baking dishes. Add the wine and garlic. Dot each shell with one-fourth of the butter. Combine the remaining ingredients in a bowl or blender and rub or whirl to a paste. Crumble over the shrimps. Bake at 350 °F (175 °C) for 10 minutes. Serve warm.

Yield: 4 servings
Exchange, 1 serving: 2 lean meat
½ bread
Calories, 1 serving: 120
Carbohydrates, 1 serving: 7 g

Lobster Tails

Seafood is certainly among the foods lowest in calories and lobster and rock lobster tails are delicious examples. You can buy lobsters alive or fresh-frozen. Live lobsters should be active and greenish in color. The lobster changes to red when cooked.

½ lb.   *lobster tail for each person*   *250 g*

Cook lobster tails in boiling, salted water for 5 minutes. Reduce heat and simmer 10 minutes longer. Check for doneness by straightening each tail. When done, the tail snaps back into a curled position; avoid overcooking. Serve warm or cold.

Yield: 1 serving
Exchange, 1 serving: 1 lean meat
Calories, 1 serving: 53
Carbohydrates, 1 serving: negligible

Lobster Thermidor

2 lbs.	live lobsters	1 kg
¼ lb.	snow-capped mushrooms, sliced	125 g
¼ c.	onion, finely chopped	60 mL
2 T.	low-calorie margarine	30 mL
2 T.	sherry	30 mL
1 T.	parsley, snipped	15 mL
½ t.	salt	2 mL
¼ t.	black pepper, freshly ground	1 mL
dash	paprika	dash
1 c.	skim milk	250 mL
2 T.	all-purpose flour	30 mL
2 T.	bread crumbs	30 mL
1 T.	Parmesan cheese, grated	15 mL

Heat 3 qts. (3 L) salted water to the boiling point. Plunge lobsters into the water, cover, and reheat to the boil. Reduce heat and simmer for 5 minutes. Remove and cool the lobsters. Carefully separate the meat from the shells; reserve the shells. Cut the lobster meat into small pieces; set aside. In a saucepan, sauté the mushrooms and onion in margarine until the onion is tender. Stir in the sherry, parsley, salt, pepper, and paprika. Combine the milk and flour in a shaker or bowl and blend thoroughly.

Add to the mushroom mixture in the saucepan. Cook and stir over low heat until the mixture thickens slightly. Remove from heat. Fold in the lobster meat. Return to the heat, and heat thoroughly. Place the empty lobster shells on a cookie sheet and fill them with the hot mixture. Combine the bread crumbs and cheese; sprinkle over the lobster mixture. Bake at 450 °F (230 °C) for 8 to 10 minutes. Serve warm.

Yield: 4 servings
Exchange, 1 serving: 2 lean meat
²/₃ bread
Calories, 1 serving: 155
Carbohydrates, 1 serving: 10 g

Lobster a la Newburg

This dish is excellent served over hot toast or croutons, or spooned into homemade Pastry Shells.

1¼ lbs.	lobster meat	500 g
2 T.	unsalted butter	30 mL
1½ c.	Madeira	375 mL
1½ c.	skim evaporated milk	375 mL
3	egg yolks, beaten	3
½ t.	salt	2 mL
⅛ t.	cayenne pepper	½ mL

Cut lobster into large serving pieces. Melt butter in a nonstick skillet. Sauté lobster over low heat for 5 minutes. Add the Madeira and simmer until liquid is almost completely evaporated. Beat the milk and egg yolks together until well blended. Add the lobster to the milk mixture and fold to blend. Return to the skillet and cook over low heat until thickened, stirring constantly. Serve warm.

Yield: 8 servings
Exchange, 1 serving: 2 lean meat
²/₃ bread
Calories, 1 serving: 153
Carbohydrates, 1 serving: 10 g

Shrimp a la Berto

A lovely shrimp dish developed by Berto of Minneapolis.

¼ lb.	jumbo shrimps	125 g
1 T.	unsalted butter	15 mL
½	garlic clove, minced	½
2 t.	parsley, minced	10 mL
¼ t.	fresh tarragon leaves, minced	1 mL
2 T.	white wine	30 mL

Split the shrimps down their backs and remove the veins. Flatten shrimps with the bottom of a glass. Arrange in a baking shell or small serving dish. Melt butter in a small nonstick skillet. Add the garlic, parsley, and tarragon and stir over low heat for 30 seconds; spread over the shrimps. Pour wine into shell. Bake at 400 °F (200 °C) for 8 minutes. Serve hot.

Yield: 1 serving
Exchange: 1 medium-fat meat
          2 fat
Calories: 171
Carbohydrates: 1 g

Sweet-and-Sour Shrimp

. . . with a delicate cherry sauce.

3 T.	cornstarch	45 mL
½ t.	fresh ginger, grated	2 mL
½ t.	salt	2 mL
1 lb.	cooked medium shrimps	500 g
	vegetable oil for frying	
1 recipe	Sweet-and-Sour Cherry Sauce, heated	1 recipe

Combine cornstarch, ginger, and salt in a shaker or plastic bag. Add the shrimps, a few at a time, and shake to coat. In a deep-fryer, heat the oil to 365 °F (184 °C); fry the shrimps until golden brown. Drain on paper towels. Divide the shrimps among 4 heated serving dishes. Cover with the heated sauce. Serve with hot mustard.

Yield: 4 servings
Exchange, 1 serving: 2 lean meat
                    ½ fruit
                    ¼ bread
Calories, 1 serving: 154
Carbohydrates, 1 serving: 10 g

Grilled Jumbo Shrimp

2 lbs.	jumbo shrimps, unshelled	1 kg
1	garlic clove, minced	1
¼ c.	lime juice, freshly squeezed	60 mL
2 T.	white wine vinegar	30 mL
	PAM nonstick vegetable cooking spray	

Split each shrimp shell on the underside down to the tail. Place shrimps in a large bowl and cover with the remaining ingredients. Fold to completely coat the shrimps. Refrigerate for 2 to 3 hours; shake or mix occasionally. Push shrimp onto 4 wooden skewers. Coat with the spray. Place over charcoal on a gas barbecue grill about 6 in. (15 cm) from low heat. Broil for 15 minutes, turning occasionally. Serve hot.

Yield: 4 servings
Exchange, 1 serving: 3 lean meat
Calories, 1 serving: 142
Carbohydrates, 1 serving: 2 g

Scallops de Anna

Tasty scallops sautéed with mushrooms in wine sauce.

	PAM nonstick vegetable cooking spray	
½ c.	onions, chopped	125 mL
1 c.	mushrooms	250 mL
2 c.	bay scallops	500 mL
¼ c.	chablis	60 mL
1 T.	cold water	15 mL
1 t.	cornstarch	5 mL

Spray a nonstick skillet with the spray. Sauté the onions and mushrooms over low heat until slightly soft. Add the scallops and chablis, cover, and simmer for 4 to 5 minutes. Blend the water and cornstarch. Slowly add to the skillet, stirring gently to avoid breaking the scallops and cook over low heat until the mixture is clear and liquid is reduced by half. Serve hot. (Tomato Pasta is a nice accompaniment for this dish.)

Yield: 4 servings
Exchange, 1 serving: 1½ lean meat
*　　　　　　　　　1 vegetable*
Calories, 1 serving: 112
Carbohydrates, 1 serving: 4 g

Bay Scallops

In this dish, scallops are cooked with snow peas, mushrooms, and ginger.

12	*large snow peas*	12
½ lb.	*mushrooms*	250 g
2 T.	*unsalted butter*	30 mL
2 c.	*bay scallops*	500 mL
3 T.	*dry white wine*	45 mL
¼ t.	*ground ginger*	1 mL
	salt and freshly ground pepper	

Clean and dice the snow peas and mushrooms. Melt half the butter in a skillet. Add the snow peas and mushrooms and sauté for 2 minutes. Stir in the scallops and wine. Cover and simmer for 3 minutes. Uncover and add the remaining butter and ginger. Simmer, uncovered, until liquid evaporates. Season with salt and pepper to taste. Serve warm.

Yield: 4 servings
Exchange, 1 serving: 2 medium-fat meat
*   1 vegetable*
Calories, 1 serving: 163
Carbohydrates, 1 serving: 4 g

Crepes aux Crevettes

2 T.	*celery, finely diced*	30 mL
2 T.	*leek bulb, finely diced*	30 mL
2 T.	*green pepper, finely diced*	30 mL
½ t.	*soy sauce*	2 mL
1 t.	*white wine*	5 mL
6-oz. bag	*Brilliant cooked frozen shrimps*	170-g bag
8	*Crepes*	8
1	*egg white, slightly beaten*	1

Place celery, leek, and green pepper in a custard cup and add 1 t. (5 mL) water. Cook on HIGH in the microwave for 30 seconds. Add soy sauce and wine. Stir to blend, cover and cool. Chop the shrimps and add the seasonings. Put an equal portion of filling on each crepe. Moisten the edges with egg white. Roll up loosely, jelly roll fashion, tucking in the edges while rolling. Place seam side down on well-greased baking sheet. Bake at 350 °F (175 °C) for 15 to 20 minutes or until crepes are browned. Serve warm.

Yield: 8 servings
Exchange, 1 serving: ½ low-fat meat
⅓ bread
Calories, 1 serving: 40
Carbohydrates, 1 serving: 4 g

Stuffed Sole Fillets

A delicious stuffing with shrimps and black olives.

Marinade:

2 T.	*lemon juice, freshly squeezed*	*30 mL*
¼ c.	*olive oil*	*60 mL*
½ c.	*dry white wine*	*125 mL*
	salt and freshly ground pepper to taste	
2¼ lbs.	*sole fillets, thinly sliced*	*1 kg*

Stuffing:

¼ c.	*bread crumbs*	*60 mL*
6-oz bag	*Brilliant cooked/frozen shrimps*	*170-g bag*
¼ c.	*black olives, pitted and chopped*	*60 mL*
1	*egg, slightly beaten*	*1*
¾ c.	*bread crumbs*	*190 mL*
	vegetable oil for frying	

Combine ingredients for the marinade in a flat baking dish and stir to blend. Clean the fish; place fish in marinade for an hour, turning occasionally. Combine the stuffing ingredients in a medium bowl; work with the back of a spoon or your hands into a semimoist mixture. Stuff each fillet; secure with a poultry pin or toothpick. Roll in the bread crumbs. Chill thoroughly. Fry in a deep oil at 375 °F (190 °C) until brown. Drain on paper towels. Serve hot.

Yield: 10 servings
Exchange, 1 serving: 1 high-fat meat
½ bread
Calories, 1 serving: 148
Carbohydrates, 1 serving: 8g

Crab on Toast Tips

Here's a favorite recipe for luncheons.

3 c	skim milk	750 mL
⅓ c.	chive, snipped in ½ in. (1.25 cm) pieces	90 mL
¼ c.	fresh parsley, snipped	60 mL
2 T	pimiento, chopped	30 mL
1 T.	fresh oregano leaves, snipped	15 mL
1 t.	salt	5 mL
	black pepper, freshly ground	
½ t.	dried basil	2 mL
3 T.	all-purpose flour	45 mL
6-oz. can	crab meat	170-g can
8	bread slices, toasted	8
	fresh parsley for garnish	

Combine 2½ c. (625 mL) milk, chive, parsley, pimiento, oregano, salt, pepper, and basil in a saucepan. Combine remaining milk and flour in shaker or bowl; blend well. Add to saucepan. Cook and stir over medium heat until very thick. Add the crab meat and heat thoroughly. Adjust the salt and pepper to taste. Serve hot over toast, garnished with a small sprig of parsley.

Yield: 8 servings
Exchange, 1 serving: 1 bread
  ½ nonfat milk
  ½ lean meat
Calories, 1 serving: 125
Carbohydrates, 1 serving: 21 g

Channel Catfish

Channel Catfish is a tasty recipe served in the best restaurants of the Midwest and along the Mississippi River.

4 (2 lbs.)	catfish, left whole	4 (1 kg)
	PAM nonstick vegetable cooking spray	
¼ c.	unsalted butter, melted	60 mL
2 T.	dry white wine	30 mL
1½ t.	salt	7 mL
1 t. of each	fresh celery, chopped	5 mL of each
	fresh sweet marjoram, chopped	
	fresh peppermint, chopped	

	fresh smooth-leaf parsley, chopped	
	fresh chervil, chopped	
	fresh thyme, chopped	
½ t.	ground paprika	2 mL

Clean the fish. Heat the barbecue to MEDIUM HOT or charcoals should be nicely white. Spray the grill surface with coating. Combine the wine, salt, vegetables, and herbs with melted butter and stir to blend. Brush one side of the catfish with the butter mixture. Set on the grill, buttered side down. Brush the catfish top with the mixture. Cook for 8 to 10 minutes on each side, occasionally brushing with the butter mixture. Serve hot.

Yield: 4 servings
Exchange, 1 serving: 3½ medium-fat meat
Calories, 1 serving: 253
Carbohydrates, 1 serving: negligible

Grilled Halibut

A colorful dish with fresh tomato sauce.

Sauce:

3	large fresh tomatoes	3
¼ c.	dry red wine	60 mL
1 T.	white vinegar	15 mL
4	garlic cloves, minced	4
1 T.	ground rosemary	15 mL
1 t.	ground thyme	5 mL
	salt and freshly ground pepper to taste	
8 (2 lbs.)	halibut steaks	8 (1 kg)
¼ c.	butter, melted	60 mL

To make the sauce, peel and cut tomatoes in chunks. Combine tomatoes with remaining sauce ingredients in a saucepan. Cook and stir over medium heat until sauce thickens. Butter fish on both sides. Place fish over medium-hot coals. Grill for about 7 minutes per side or until meat becomes opaque. Arrange fish on a heated serving plate or platter and top with the tomato sauce. Serve hot.

Yield: 8 servings
Exchange, 1 serving: 2¼ medium-fat meat
Calories, 1 serving: 164
Carbohydrates, 1 serving: 2 g

Smoked Fillet of Salmon

Salmon is appetizing when baked with Monterey Jack cheese.

1 lb.	smoked salmon fillets	500 g
1 T.	butter	15 mL
2	garlic cloves, minced	2
1½ oz.	Monterey Jack cheese	45 g

Place salmon fillets on an ovenproof plate or platter. Combine butter and garlic and heat in a microwave until hot. With a brush, coat the fillets with the garlic butter. Bake at 350 °F (175 °C) for 15 minutes. Meanwhile, slice cheese into 8 thin slices (or enough for the number of fillets you have). Place a cheese slice on each fillet; continue baking 10 minutes longer or until cheese melts. Serve immediately.

Yield: 8 servings
Exchange, 1 serving: 2 medium-fat meat
Calories, 1 serving: 149
Carbohydrates, 1 serving: negligible

Fish Florentine

2¼ lbs.	fish fillets	1 kg
3 lbs.	fresh spinach	1.5 kg
2 T.	low-calorie margarine	30 mL
1½ T.	all-purpose flour	22 mL
½ t.	salt	2 mL
¼ t.	black pepper, freshly ground	1 mL
1½ c.	skim milk	375 mL
½ c.	sharp cheddar cheese, grated	125 mL

Wash and clean the fillets and set aside. Thoroughly wash the spinach. Place spinach in a saucepan, cover and cook over low heat (do not add water). When spinach is just tender, drain, and coarsely chop. Place spinach in a baking dish. Melt margarine in a saucepan; blend in the flour, salt, and pepper. Slowly stir in the milk; stir and cook until thickened. Add the cheese; heat until cheese melts. Pour sauce over the spinach. Lay the fillets on top and bake at 375 °F (190 °C) for 30 minutes. Serve hot.

Yield: 8 servings
Exchange, 1 serving: 1 high-fat meat
½ vegetable
Calories, 1 serving: 129
Carbohydrates, 1 serving: 8 g

Florets of Shark

1 lb.	shark steak	500 g
1 T.	unsalted butter	15 mL
3	whole cloves	3
1	bay leaf	1
1 T.	fresh parsley	15 mL
¼ c.	onion, chopped	60 mL
¼ c.	cream sherry	60 mL
1 t.	lemon juice	5 mL
1 t.	soy sauce	5 mL

Carefully cut the skin and bones from the shark steak. Cut out the flower design on each side of the steak to make florets. Meanwhile, melt the butter in a nonstick skillet. Add the cloves, bay leaf, parsley, and onion; sauté for 3 minutes. Add the shark florets. Sauté until fish turns white on both sides. Add the remaining ingredients. Cover and simmer for 20 to 30 minutes. Serve hot on a bed of blanched spinach, if desired.

Yield: 2 servings
Exchange, 1 serving: 2 medium-fat meat
Calories, 1 serving: 162
Carbohydrates, 1 serving: 2 g

Orange Roughy Napa Valley

Orange roughy is a fish from Australia.

½ lb.	orange roughy	250 g
¼ c.	Napa Valley Rhine wine	60 mL
3	white onion slices, cut in rings	3
2 T.	lemon juice	30 mL
2 T.	fresh chive	30 mL
1 t.	fresh basil	5 mL
	salt and pepper to taste	

Wash and clean the fish. Place in a single layer in a well-greased baking dish. Cover with remaining ingredients. Bake uncovered at 400 °F (200 °C) for 20 minutes. Serve hot.

Yield: 2 servings
Exchange, 1 serving: 2 lean meat
Calories, 1 serving: 129
Carbohydrates, 1 serving: 3 g

Sauerbraten

The famous marinated beef with a light herb gravy.

2¼ lbs. lean beef shoulder roast   1 kg

Marinade:

1	onion, cut in rings	1
4	peppercorns	4
2	whole cloves	2
1	bay leaf	1
1¼ c.	vinegar	310 mL
1½ c.	water	375 mL

For cooking:

2 T.	vegetable oil	30 mL
1 t.	salt	5 ml
1¼ c.	hot water	310 mL
2 t.	cornstarch	10 mL
1 T.	cold water	15 mL

Wash and drain the beef. Place in a suitable container or large bowl. To marinate, add the onion rings and spices; cover with the vinegar and water; refrigerate for 4 to 6 days, turning the meat once a day. Remove beef from marinade and pat dry with paper towels. Heat the oil in a skillet. Quickly brown the beef on both sides; reduce the heat. Salt the meat and carefully add the hot water to the pan. Cover and simmer for 1½ hours; add extra water, if needed. Remove the beef to a warm platter. To thicken the gravy, blend cornstarch and cold water; stir into the liquid in the skillet and cook until smooth and thickened. Pour over the beef or serve separately in a sauceboat.

Yield: 6 servings
Exchange, 1 serving: 3 high-fat meat
Calories, 1 serving: 308
Carbohydrates, 1 serving: negligible

Corned Beef and Cabbage

In true Irish fashion, this dish should be served with whole new potatoes.

2¼ lbs.	lean, boneless corned beef	1 kg
1	large cabbage	1
	salt and pepper to taste	

Place beef in a Dutch oven; cover with water and simmer for 3 hours.

Clean and core the cabbage; cut into eighths. Add to the Dutch oven with additional water, if needed. Simmer until the cabbage is tender. Serve warm.

Yield: 8 servings
Exchange, 1 serving: 2 lean meat
1 vegetable
Calories, 1 serving: 144
Carbohydrates, 1 serving: 4 g

Beef with Broccoli

| ½ lb. | beef, thinly sliced | 250 g |

Marinade:

1 t.	cornstarch	5 mL
2 t.	soy sauce	10 mL
2 t.	sherry	10 mL

For cooking:

1 qt.	fresh broccoli, florets and stems	1 L
2 T.	vegetable oil	30 mL
1 c.	Chicken Stock	250 mL
1	fresh ginger wedge	1
2 t.	cornstarch	10 mL
1 T.	cold water	15 mL

Place beef in a container or bowl. Combine ingredients for the marinade and blend until the cornstarch dissolves. Pour over the beef and fold or flip the slices to coat them. Marinate in the refrigerator for at least 2 hours. Slice broccoli stems diagonally into paper-thin slices. Heat a wok or skillet over high heat; add half of the oil. When hot, add the broccoli and stir-fry for 30 seconds. Stir in the chicken stock, cover, lower heat and cook for 5 minutes. Remove the broccoli and stock. Drain the beef thoroughly. Reheat the wok and add the remaining oil. When the oil is hot, add the beef and stir-fry for 50 seconds. Return broccoli mixture to the wok. Blend the cornstarch and water; stir into the wok and cook until the sauce thickens.

Yield: 4 servings
Exchange, 1 serving: 2 medium-fat meat
1½ vegetable
1 fat
Calories, 1 serving: 199
Carbohydrates, 1 serving: 8 g

Chateaubriand

Broiled beef tenderloin with homemade Chateaubriand Sauce makes a tasty dish.

3 slices	bacon	3 slices
1-lb.	beef tenderloin (one thick slice)	500-g
1 recipe	Chateaubriand Sauce	1 recipe

Cut bacon slices in half. Lay 3 of the bacon pieces on each side of the beef. Using toothpicks, pin to the tenderloin. Broil to the desired doneness. Remove and discard the bacon. Place tenderloin on a heated serving platter. Slice tenderloin diagonally across the grain into thin slices. Cover with hot Chateaubriand Sauce. Serve immediately.

Yield: 5 servings
Exchange, 1 serving: 2 medium-fat meat
Calories, 1 serving: 157
Carbohydrates, 1 serving: 1 g

Sirloin Pepper Steak

Sautéed with peppercorns and white grape sauce, this steak is quick to cook. But if you like your meat well done, this is not the recipe for you.

1 T.	peppercorns, cracked	15 mL
1½ lbs.	sirloin steak, thickly cut	750 g
60	white seedless grapes	60
½ c.	water	125 mL
1 t.	cornstarch	5 mL

Press the cracked peppercorns into both sides of the steak. Cover and rest at room temperature for 45 to 60 minutes. In a large nonstick skillet over medium heat, cook the steak to desired doneness. (The best method is to fry until both sides are dark brown; the meat in the middle will be pink to light red.) Place steak on a heated serving platter. Add the grapes to juices in the skillet and sauté for 2 minutes. Combine the water and cornstarch and stir to blend. Pour into the skillet and cook, stirring constantly, until the mixture thickens slightly. Pour over the steak. Serve hot.

Yield: 6 servings
Exchange, 1 serving: 2 lean meat
²/₃ fruit
Calories, 1 serving: 136
Carbohydrates, 1 serving: 6 g

Beef Stroganoff

I adapted the classic recipe for the diabetic diet.

1 lb.	beef sirloin fillet	500 g
2 T.	unsalted butter	30 mL
1	large yellow onion, chopped	1
½ lb.	snow-white mushrooms, sliced	250 g
½ t.	glace-de-viande	2 mL
1 c.	Beef Stock	250 mL
2 t.	cornstarch	10 mL
1 t.	salt	5 mL
1 t.	black pepper, freshly ground	5 mL
1 c.	low-fat yogurt	250 mL

Trim the beef fillets of any fat; cut across grain into 2-in. (5-cm) by ½-in. (1.30-cm) strips. Heat the butter in a skillet until bubbles appear; brown the meat. Remove beef strips with a slotted spoon and place on a well-greased casserole. In the same skillet, sauté the onions and mushrooms until tender. Remove vegetables with a slotted spoon and place on the beef strips in the casserole. Stir glace-de-viande into the skillet and remove from the heat. Blend the beef stock and cornstarch until smooth; stir into the mixture in the skillet. Return to the heat and stir until sauce begins to boil. Add salt and pepper. Stir in the yogurt, a little at a time, until well blended. Pour over beef and vegetables in casserole. Cover and bake at 375 °F (190 °C) for 30 minutes or until thoroughly heated. Serve hot.

Yield: 8 servings
Exchange, 1 serving: 2 lean meat
1 vegetable
Calories, 1 serving: 133
Carbohydrates, 1 serving: 4 g

Fruity Baby Beef Liver

Liver is delicious with white grapes and mandarin orange sauce.

2	bacon slices	2
½ lb.	baby beef liver	250 g
4 T.	all-purpose flour	60 mL
2	parsnips, thinly sliced	2
11-oz. can	mandarin oranges in light syrup	311-g can
40	white seedless grapes	40

In a skillet, fry the bacon until crisp; set aside. Pour half of the fat into a small bowl and reserve for the cooking. Cut the liver into large bite-size pieces. Put half of the flour in a plastic bag; add half of the liver and shake to coat the liver. Fry liver in the hot bacon fat over high heat until browned. Remove liver and set aside. Pour reserved fat into the skillet. Repeat, shaking the remaining flour and liver in the bag. Fry the liver and remove from the skillet. Add the parsnips, oranges with the syrup, and the grapes to the skillet. Cover and simmer for 4 minutes. Return liver to the skillet. Crumble bacon and add to the liver. Simmer, uncovered, until liver is hot. Serve immediately. (This recipe may be served over pasta or rice.)

Yield: 6 servings
Exchange, 1 serving: 1 medium-fat meat
1½ fruit
Calories, 1 serving: 125
Carbohydrates, 1 serving: 15 g

Meat Tortellini with Medley Sauce

2 c.	skim milk	500 mL
½ c.	broccoli, chopped	125 mL
½ c.	cauliflower, chopped	125 mL
1 c.	snow-capped mushrooms, sliced	250 mL
¼ c.	white onion, chopped	60 mL
¼ c.	cold water	60 mL
2 T.	all-purpose flour	30 mL
2 12-oz. pkg.	meat-filled tortellini	2 310-g pkg.

To make the Medley Sauce, combine the milk and vegetables in top of a double boiler. Cook over simmering water until vegetables are al dente. Combine water and flour in a shaker or bowl and blend thoroughly; pour into the vegetable mixture. Cook and stir until slightly thickened (do not boil or milk may curdle). Continue cooking to desired thickness. Meanwhile, cook the tortellini; drain. Serve Medley Sauce over tortellini. Garnish with parsley sprigs. Serve hot.

Yield: 6 servings
Exchange, 1 serving: 2 bread
2 vegetable
Calories, 1 serving: 190
Carbohydrates, 1 serving: 40 g

Crown Pork Roast

Crown roast with a sweet stuffing.

4½ lbs.	*lean pork loin*	*2 kg*
½ c.	*orange jucie*	*125 mL*
¼ c.	*diatetic mint jelly*	*60 mL*
¾ c.	*water*	*190 mL*
2 c.	*dry bread crumbs*	*500 mL*
½ c.	*onions, chopped*	*125 mL*
½ c.	*celery, chopped*	*125 mL*
2 T.	*fresh parsley, snipped*	*30 mL*
2 t.	*dried sage, crumbled*	*10 mL*
1 t.	*salt*	*5 mL*
¼ t.	*black pepper, freshly ground*	*1 mL*

Have the butcher trim and cut the bone away from the loin; slice into 12 chops from the fat side to the back. Twist the loin into a crown shape and secure with string. Combine the orange juice, jelly, and water in a saucepan. Heat just enough to melt the jelly. Stir in the remaining ingredients to make a moist stuffing; add extra water, if needed. Place roast on a meat rack in a roasting pan. Spoon the stuffing into the middle of the pork crown. Roast at 325 °F (165 °C) for 2 to 2½ hours or until the pork is tender, basting occasionally with the pan juices. Serve on a heated platter.

Yield: 12 servings
Exchange, 1 serving: 3½ high-fat meat
1 bread
Calories, 1 serving: 425
Carbohydrates, 1 serving: 13 g

French Pork Loin

Use boneless pork loin for this recipe.

½ lb. (4)	pork loin, French-cut very thinly	500 g (4)
2	bread slices, crusts removed	2
4 large	snow-capped mushrooms	4 large
¼ c.	chive, snipped	60 mL
	salt and freshly ground pepper to taste	

Remove excess fat from the pork, making sure not to break the meat. Combine bread and mushrooms in a food processor or blender and blend into a paste. Spoon into a bowl. Stir in the chive, salt, and pepper. Shape the stuffing into 4 equal finger-like forms. Place in middle of each pork slice. Fold ends over the stuffing and secure meat with a poultry pin or toothpick. Grill over medium-hot coals for 15 to 20 minutes until thoroughly cooked. Serve hot.

Yield: 4 servings
Exchange, 1 serving: 1 high-fat meat
½ bread
Calories, 1 serving: 142
Carbohydrates, 1 serving: 8 g

Baked Iowa Chops

An Iowa chop is a type of cut from the pork loin.

1½ lbs. (4)	pork loin chops	750 g (4)
	PAM nonstick vegetable cooking spray	
½ c.	corn bread crumbs	125 mL
1 t.	salt	5 mL
½ t.	black pepper, freshly ground	2 mL
1	egg white	1

Have the butcher cut a slit pocket in each chop. Spray a nonstick skillet with the spray. Brown the chops on both sides over low heat (do not crowd pan). Combine the remaining ingredients in a bowl; stir to blend and add enough water to make a moist stuffing. Stuff into pocket in the chops. Secure with small skewers or toothpicks. Place chops in a baking pan. Add ½ c. (125 mL) water to the pan. Season with salt and pepper to taste. Cover. Bake at 350 °F (175 °C) for an hour or until the meat is well browned and tender. Serve immediately on a heated platter or plates.

Yield: 4 servings
Exchange, 1 serving: 3¼ high-fat meat
1 bread
Calories, 1 serving: 391
Carbohydrates, 1 serving: 14 g

Split Pork Ribs with Tangerine Sauce

4 (¾ lb.)	split pork ribs	4 (375 g)
1 recipe	Tangerine Sauce	1 recipe

Place ribs on a grill over medium-hot coals. Grill for 15 minutes; turn and grill the second side for 15 minutes. Brush sauce on topside of the ribs; brush with sauce and turn every 5 minutes until done.

Yield: 4 servings
Exchange, 1 serving: 1½ high-fat meat
Calories, 1 serving: 160
Carbohydrates, 1 serving: negligible

Smoked Picnic Shoulder

A zesty recipe with mustard, vinegar, and homemade jelly.

4½ lbs.	uncooked smoked picnic shoulder	2 kg
1 c.	Red Currant Jelly	250 mL
2 t.	pommery mustard	10 mL
2 t.	white wine vinegar	10 mL
1 env.	Equal low-calorie sweetener	1 env.

Place the picnic shoulder in a large Dutch oven; cover with water and bring to the boil. Reduce heat, cover, and simmer for 2½ to 3 hours or until tender. With 2 meat forks, lift the shoulder and place on a heat-proof platter. Broil about 5 in. (2 cm) from the heat until the surface is lightly browned. Meanwhile, combine the jelly, mustard, and vinegar in a saucepan. Heat just to the boiling point and until the jelly melts. Remove from the heat. When the saucepan is cool enough to place your hand directly on the bottom, stir in the sweetener. Serve the sauce with the cooked picnic shoulder.

Yield: 24 servings
Exchange, 1 serving: 2½ high-fat meat
Calories, 1 serving: 270
Carbohydrates, 1 serving: negligible

Loin of Pork with Burgundy Sauce

2¼ lbs.	boneless pork loin	1 kg
½ c.	Burgundy	125 mL
1 T.	Burgundy wine vinegar	15 mL
2 t.	cornstarch	10 mL
1 t.	lemon juice, freshly squeezed	5 mL
2 t.	liquid fructose	10 mL

Place loin, fat side up, on a rack in a baking dish. Bake at 325 °F (165 °C) for 2 hours. Blend the Burgundy, wine vinegar, cornstarch, and lemon juice in a small saucepan. Cook over low heat until the mixture thickens and is reduced by half. Remove from heat; stir in the fructose. Just before serving, pour over the pork. Serve warm.

Yield: 12 servings
Exchange, 1 serving: 2 medium-fat meat
¼ bread
Calories, 1 serving: 180
Carbohydrates, 1 serving: 3 g

Stuffed Pork Chops with Maple-Orange Sauce

6 (2 lbs.)	pork chops	6 (1 kg)
1 c.	celery, chopped	250 mL
1 c.	snow-capped mushrooms, sliced	250 mL
½ c.	onion, chopped	125 mL
2 T.	unsalted butter	30 mL
1 t.	salt	5 mL
½ t.	poultry seasoning	2 mL
¼ t.	black pepper, freshly ground	1 mL
1 c.	dietetic maple syrup	250 mL
½ c.	orange juice	125 mL

Chill the pork chops in the freezer until firm on sides but not completely frozen. Cut a pocket in each chop. In a nonstick skillet, sauté the celery, mushrooms, and onions in the butter for 5 minutes; remove from heat. Add the salt, poultry seasoning, and pepper; stir to blend. Cool slightly. Spoon mixture into the pocket in each chop. Over low heat, brown the chops in the skillet without crowding them. Pour the mixture of syrup and orange juice over the chops in the skillet. Cover skillet and simmer for 20 minutes. Remove cover and simmer about 10 more minutes, or until juices have evaporated to half and chops are nicely glazed, basting frequently with the pan juices. Serve hot.

Yield: 6 servings
Exchange, 1 serving: 4 medium-fat meat
½ bread
Calories, 1 serving: 320
Carbohydrates, 1 serving: 8 g

Southern-Style Baked Fresh Ham

Although seldom seen on menus in the North, this ham recipe is a favorite in the South.

4½ lbs.	fresh ham	2 kg
3	bay leaves	3
1	fresh red chili, diced	1
1	apple, finely chopped	1
1	cinnamon stick	1
2 T.	salt	30 mL
3 T.	Dijon-style mustard	45 mL
1 t.	Worcestershire sauce	5 mL
¼ t.	ground cloves	1 mL

Place ham in a large kettle or Dutch oven. Cover with boiling water; add the bay leaves, chili, apple, cinnamon, and salt; cover and simmer for 2 hours. Remove ham from kettle and chill; refrigerate the broth. The next day, remove rind and fat from the ham. Remove the congealed fat from surface of broth. Combine mustard, Worcestershire sauce, and cloves in a small bowl; stir to blend. Spread on the surface of the ham. Place ham on a rack in a baking pan. Pour broth into the pan. Bake at 300 °F (150 °C) for 2 to 3 hours, basting occasionally with the drippings in the baking pan. Add more water, if needed. Serve hot.

Yield: 24 servings
Exchange, 1 serving: 2 medium-fat meat
Calories, 1 serving: 143
Carbohydrates, 1 serving: negligible

German-Style Chops with Sauerkraut

6 (1½ lbs.)	pork chops, thinly sliced	6 (750 g)
1 qt.	sauerkraut, drained	1 L
1 c.	dry white wine	250 mL
1 c.	water	250 mL
1	onion, chopped	1
8	peppercorns	8
2 T.	caraway seed	30 mL
1 T.	granulated sugar replacement	15 mL

Arrange pork chops on bottom of a well-greased, large and deep skillet. Spread sauerkraut over the chops. Combine the remaining ingredients and pour over the sauerkraut. Cover and simmer for an hour. Drain thoroughly before serving. Serve warm.

Yield: 6 servings
Exchange, 1 serving: 2⅓ high-fat meat
1 vegetable
Calories, 1 serving: 268
Carbohydrates, 1 serving: 6 g

Pork Tenderloin in Yogurt

1 lb.	pork tenderloin	500 g
1 T.	vegetable oil	15 mL
1 c.	Dannon plain low-fat yogurt	250 mL
2 t.	all-purpose flour	10 mL

Cut the tenderloin into 1-in. (2.5-cm) slices. Brown tenderloin in oil in a nonstick skillet. Cover with the yogurt and simmer for 20 minutes. Remove meat to heated platter. With a whisk, blend the flour with the sauce in the skillet and simmer for 3 minutes. Pour sauce over the hot meat. Serve hot.

Yield: 6 servings
Exchange, 1 serving: 2½ medium-fat meat
Calories, 1 serving: 187
Carbohydrates, 1 serving: negligible

Pepper Venison Tenderloin

1 lb.	venison tenderloin, cut into 4 thick slices	500 g
2 t.	black peppercorns, crushed	10 mL
¼ c.	red wine vinegar	60 mL
1¼ c.	unsweetened grapefruit juice	375 mL
¼ c.	fresh oregano leaves, chopped, or	60 mL
	2 t. (10 mL) dried oregano, crushed	
2	bay leaves, crushed	2

Butterfly the tenderloin slices. To butterfly the venison, cut each thick slice lengthwise, almost in half, leaving a meat hinge; open up to resemble a butterfly (or have your butcher butterfly the meat for you). Rub with crushed pepper. Place in a flat glass baking dish or container; marinate for 2 hours. Combine the remaining ingredients and pour over the tenderloin. Marinate at least 5 hours or overnight in the refrigerator. Remove meat from the marinade. Brush off excess pepper mix. Place tenderloin slices over medium-hot coals for 7 to 10 minutes per side or to the desired doneness. Serve hot on heated plates.

Yield: 4 servings
Exchange, 1 serving: 2 medium-fat meat
Calories, 1 serving: 143
Carbohydrates, 1 serving: negligible

Braised Venison Chops

6 (2 oz. each)	venison chops	6 (60 g each)
2 T.	soy sauce	30 mL
1 t.	Dijon-style mustard	5 mL

Place chops in a single layer in a shallow baking pan. Combine the soy sauce and mustard in a small bowl; stir to blend completely. Pour sauce over the chops; marinate at least 5 hours at room temperature or overnight in the refrigerator. Coat a nonstick skillet with oil. Brown the chops on both sides. Reduce the heat, add the remaining marinade, and cover the pan. Continue cooking until chops are the desired doneness; about 15 minutes are needed for medium-rare chops. Serve warm.

Yield: 6 servings
Exchange, 1 serving: 1 medium-fat meat
Calories, 1 serving: 71
Carbohydrates, 1 serving: negligible

Supreme Venison

Venison is marinated in red wine before roasting.

3 lbs.	venison roast	1½ kg
1 c.	Burgundy	250 mL
1 c.	water	250 mL
1 t.	salt	5 mL
2	bay leaves	2
8	whole cloves	8
6	thyme leaves, torn	6
3	whole allspice	3
1 slice	bacon	1 slice

Place venison in a deep bowl. Combine the Burgundy, water, salt, bay leaves, cloves, thyme, and allspice and pour over the venison. Cover and marinate for 3 days in the refrigerator. Drain and reserve the marinade. Pat the venison until dry. In a skillet, fry the bacon until crisp. Drain and crumble the bacon. Add the venison to the hot bacon fat and brown on both sides. Stir in ¾ c. (190 mL) of the reserved marinade and the crumbled bacon. Reduce heat, cover, and simmer for 2 to 3 hours or until the venison is tender; add extra marinade, if needed. Serve hot.

Yield: 10 servings
Exchange, 1 serving: 2 medium-fat meat
Calories, 1 serving: 171
Carbohydrates, 1 serving: negligible

Herbed Lamb

Cubes of lamb are braised in herb wine for a special dish.

2 lbs.	boneless lamb loin	1 kg
1 T.	olive oil	15 mL
1 c.	onion, chopped	250 mL
2 T.	carrot, finely chopped	30 mL
2	garlic cloves, minced	2
1	bay leaf	1
6	fresh thyme leaves, torn	6
4	fresh sage leaves, torn	4
1 c.	Rhine wine	250 mL
	salt and freshly ground pepper to taste	

Cut the lamb into 1-in. (2.5-cm) cubes. Heat the oil in nonstick skillet; brown the lamb cubes. Add the onion, carrot, garlic, bay leaf, thyme, and sage to the skillet. Cook and stir for 1 minute. Add the wine and heat to the boiling point; reduce the heat, cover skillet, and simmer for about 1½ hours or until the lamb is tender.

Yield: 10 servings
Exchange, 1 serving: 2 lean meat
Calories, 1 serving: 122
Carbohydrates, 1 serving: negligible

Stuffed Breast of Lamb

2 lbs.	*breast of lamb*	*1 kg*
2 c.	*cooked long-grain rice*	*500 mL*
1 T.	*lemon rind, grated*	*15 mL*
2-oz. can	*flat anchovy fillets, drained and chopped*	*60-g can*
½ c.	*fresh parsley, chopped*	*125 mL*
1	*egg, beaten*	*1*
½ t.	*black pepper, freshly ground*	*2 mL*

Cut a pocket in the lamb breast for the stuffing. To make the stuffing, combine the remaining ingredients and mix well; stuff into the lamb pocket. Secure with toothpicks or poultry pins. Place on a roasting rack in a shallow baking pan. Bake at 350 °F (175 °C) for 2 hours, basting occasionally with pan drippings.

Yield: 10 servings
Exchange, 1 serving: 2 medium-fat meat
*   ⅔ bread*
Calories, 1 serving: 204
Carbohydrates, 1 serving: 10 g

Lamb Steaks Baked with Orange Ginger Sauce

2 (½ lb.)	*lamb steaks*	*2 (500 g)*
1 t.	*salt*	*5 mL*
2	*medium oranges*	*2*
1 T.	*brown sugar replacement*	*15 mL*
½ t.	*ground ginger*	*5 mL*
¼ t.	*ground cloves*	*1 mL*
4	*fresh mint leaves*	*4*

Lay the lamb steak in a shallow baking pan. Slice oranges with the rind; lay on top of the steak. Combine the remaining ingredients and sprinkle over the lamb and oranges. Cover and bake at 325 °F (165 °C) for 35 to 40 minutes, basting occasionally with pan juices.

Yield: 2 servings
Exchange, 1 serving: 1¾ high-fat meat
½ fruit
Calories, 1 serving: 219
Carbohydrates, 1 serving: 5g

Veal Birds

2 slices	bread, crusts removed	2 slices
¼ c.	leek, finely chopped	60 mL
½ t.	ground thyme	2 mL
¼ t.	ground basil	1 mL
½ lb.	veal shoulder steak, cut into 4 thin slices	250 g

Break or cut the bread into small pieces. Combine the pieces, leek, thyme, and basil in a food processor or bowl; work until completely blended. Place one-fourth of bread mixture on each veal slice and carefully roll up; secure with a toothpick or poultry pin. In a nonstick skillet, brown the veal rolls on all sides; transfer to a baking pan. Rinse the skillet with a small amount of water to loosen the browned residue; pour over the rolls and cover the pan tightly. Bake at 350 °F (175 °C) for 35 to 45 minutes or until meat is tender.

Yield: 4 servings
Exchange, 1 serving: 1 medium-fat meat
½ bread
Calories, 1 serving: 106
Carbohydrates, 1 serving: 7 g

Rabbit with Fettucine

1½ lbs.	rabbit	750 g
2 T.	butter	30 mL
½ lb.	mushroom caps	250 g
1 lb.	pearl onions, cleaned	500 g
2	garlic cloves, sliced	2
2 T.	all-purpose flour	30 mL
1	bay leaf	1
1 t.	ground thyme	5 mL
2 T.	tomato paste	30 mL
1 c.	dry white wine	250 mL
1 c.	Chicken Stock	250 mL
6 c.	cooked fettucine	1.5 L

Wash, dry, and cut the rabbit into 10 serving segments. Melt the butter in a nonstick skillet. Brown the rabbit on both sides without crowding the skillet. When brown, remove the rabbit and reserve. Add the mushroom caps and onions to the skillet and sauté until mushrooms are brown. Add the garlic and cook 30 seconds. Lightly sprinkle flour over the mushrooms, onions, and garlic; cook and fold for about 3 to 4 minutes until the flour is incorporated into the mixture. Add the bay leaf and thyme. Combine the tomato paste, wine, and chicken stock in a bowl; slowly add to the vegetables, stirring to blend. Return the rabbit pieces to the skillet. Cover, reduce heat, and simmer for about 45 to 50 minutes until the rabbit is tender. Place hot fettucine on a heated platter, top with the rabbit, and cover with the sauce.

Yield: 10 servings
Exchange, 1 serving: 1½ medium-fat meat
1½ bread
Calories, 1 serving: 195
Carbohydrates, 1 serving: 21

Sesame Chicken

The toasted sesame seeds give this chicken a nutty flavor.

1	egg	1
½ c.	skim milk	125 mL
½ c.	all-purpose flour	125 mL
¼ c.	sesame seeds, toasted	60 mL
1 t.	salt	5 mL
¼ c.	Diet Fleischmann's margarine	60 mL
2¼ lbs.	frying chicken, segmented	1 kg

Combine the egg and milk in a shallow bowl; whip to completely mix. In another shallow bowl, mix the flour, toasted sesame seeds, and salt. Melt the margarine in a 13×9-in. (33×23-cm) baking pan. Dip chicken parts in the milk mixture; then roll in the flour mixture. Shake to remove any excess flour. Place chicken in the baking pan, turning once to coat sides with margarine. Bake at 350 °F (175 °C) for 1¼ hours or until chicken is crisp, brown, and tender.

Yield: 8 servings
Exchange, 1 serving: 2½ medium-fat meat
½ bread
1 fat
Calories, 1 serving: 277
Carbohydrates, 1 serving: 7 g

Pollo alla Cacciatore

2¼ lbs.	frying chicken	1 kg
2 T.	olive oil	30 mL
1	medium onion, chopped	1
1	medium green pepper, chopped	1
1 c.	red pepper, finely chopped	250 mL
2	garlic cloves, finely chopped	2
3	tomatoes, peeled and chopped	3
1½ c.	tomato sauce	375 mL
2	bay leaves	2
1 t.	salt	5 mL
1 t.	oregano	5 mL
½ t.	celery seed	2 mL
2 T.	dry white wine	30 mL

Wash and cut the chicken into serving segments. Heat the oil in large and deep skillet and brown chicken; remove and set aside. In the skillet, cook the onion, peppers, and garlic until tender and lightly browned. Add the remaining ingredients, except the wine, and blend. Simmer for 5 minutes. Return chicken to the skillet; cover and cook for 30 minutes. Uncover, add the wine and cook, uncovered, for 10 to 15 minutes or until the chicken is tender. Remove chicken to a hot serving plate. Discard bay leaves and any excess fat from the sauce and pour over the chicken. This recipe makes a tasty combination served with pasta. Serve hot.

Yield: 12 servings
Exchange, 1 serving: 2 lean meat
1 vegetable
½ fat
Calories, 1 serving: 162
Carbohydrates, 1 serving: 5 g

Almond Orange Chicken

An easy and elegant entrée.

2¼ lbs.	frying chicken, segmented	1 kg
1 t.	salt	5 mL
1 t.	paprika	5 mL
¼ t.	black pepper, freshly ground	1 mL
¼ c.	Diet Fleischmann's margarine	60 mL
1 c.	fresh orange juice	250 mL
½ c.	slivered almonds, toasted	125 mL

Wash the chicken and pat dry. Combine the salt, paprika, and pepper;

rub the spice thoroughly into the chicken. Heat the margarine in large nonstick skillet. Sauté chicken until golden on all sides. Cover, reduce heat, and cook for 25 minutes or until chicken is tender. Remove to a heated platter and place in a warm oven. Pour orange juice into the skillet and stir to loosen any browned particles; bring to the boil and cook until mixture is reduced by half. Pour over the chicken. Sprinkle with the toasted almonds. Serve hot.

Yield: 8 servings
Exchange, 1 serving: 2½ medium-fat meat
                ½ fruit
                1 fat
Calories, 1 serving: 247
Carbohydrates, 1 serving: 4 g

Coq au Vin

	PAM nonstick vegetable cooking spray	
2¼ lbs.	*frying chicken, segmented*	1 kg
8	*shallots, peeled*	8
½ c.	*carrots, coarsely shredded*	125 mL
1	*garlic clove, minced*	1
¼ lb.	*snow-capped mushrooms, sliced*	120 g
3	*parsley sprigs, chopped*	3
1 small	*bay leaf*	1 small
¼ t.	*thyme*	1 mL
2 c.	*dark red wine*	500 mL

Skillet method: Coat a nonstick skillet with the spray; slowly brown the chicken. Remove the chicken and set aside. Sauté shallots, carrots, garlic, and mushrooms in the skillet until lightly browned. Return the browned chicken to the skillet and add the remaining ingredients. Cover and simmer for 20 to 30 minutes or until chicken is tender.

Oven Method: After browning the chicken as directed above, remove chicken and place in a 2-qt. (2-L) casserole. Sauté the shallots, carrots, garlic, and mushrooms in the skillet until lightly browned. Add the remaining ingredients and cook for 3 minutes. Pour the sauce over the chicken. Cover and bake at 350 °F (175 °C) for an hour or until chicken is tender.

Yield: 12 servings
Exchange, 1 serving: 2 lean meat
                ½ vegetable
Calories, 1 serving: 133
Carbohydrates, 1 serving: 2 g

Chicken Kiev

Many people think of Chicken Kiev when they think of gourmet cooking. It is not a hard dish to prepare and it will add a touch of elegance to any meal or party.

¼ lb.	Diet Fleischmann's margarine	120 g
2 T.	fresh parsley, finely chopped	30 mL
¼ t.	garlic powder	1 mL
4 (4 oz. each)	chicken breasts, deboned and skinned	4 (120 g each)
¼ c.	all-purpose flour	60 mL
1	egg	1
1 T.	water	15 mL
½ c.	fine bread crumbs	125 mL
	vegetable oil for deep-frying	

Combine the margarine, parsley, and garlic powder in a bowl; stir to blend. Place in the freezer until slightly firm; then roll in plastic wrap to form a roll 1 in. (2.5 cm) in diameter. Freeze the roll. Surround each chicken breast with plastic wrap. Pound and flatten the chicken with a rolling pin until ¼-in. (6-mm) thick. Cut the frozen margarine roll into 4 sticks; place a stick at the edge of each chicken breast. Fold ends over and roll up jelly-roll style; press the seam to seal. Combine egg with water and beat slightly. Coat each chicken roll by dipping all sides in the flour, the egg mixture, and the bread crumbs until completely covered. Refrigerate for at least an hour. Fry the rolls in deep oil at 375 °F (190°C) for 5 to 6 minutes or until golden brown; drain. Serve hot.

Yield: 4 servings
Exchange, 1 serving: 2¾ high-fat meat
1 bread
Calories, 1 serving: 353
Carbohydrates, 1 serving: 14 g

Coq Flambé

4½ lbs.	roasting chicken	2 kg
	salt	
½ c.	brandy, warmed	125 mL
½ c.	port wine	125 mL
2 T.	skim evaporated milk	30 mL

Remove excess fat from the chicken. Rub chicken cavity and surface with salt. Place chicken in a well-greased baking pan. Brown at 425 °F

(220 °C) for 15 minutes; remove from oven. Pour brandy over the chicken and ignite; baste chicken with ignited brandy until the flames die. Combine port wine and evaporated milk and stir to blend. Pour over the chicken. Return chicken to oven, reduce heat to 325 °F (165 °C), and continue baking, basting frequently, for about an hour or until chicken is golden brown and tender.

Yield: 12 servings
Exchange, 1 serving: 3½ medium-fat meat
½ fruit
Calories, 1 serving: 285
Carbohydrates, 1 serving: 5 g

Pollo de Sevilla

A flaming chicken at the table arouses attention.

4½ lbs.	roasting chicken	2 kg
	salt	
1	carrot, sliced	1
1	leek, sliced	1
1	celery stalk, sliced	1
½ c.	white onion, chopped	125 mL
5	peppercorns	5
1	garlic clove	1
1	large bay leaf	1
1	fresh thyme sprig	1
½ c.	dry red wine	125 mL
¼ c.	brandy, warmed	60 mL

Remove excess fat from the chicken. Wash and sprinkle chicken with salt. Place chicken, breast side up, in a large baking pan. Brown for 20 minutes in a 400 °F (200 °C) oven. Remove chicken and reduce heat to 375 °F (190 °C). Add carrot, leek, celery, onion, peppercorns, garlic, bay leaf, and thyme to the pan. Pour wine and an equal amount of water over the chicken. Return to the oven and roast for 1½ hours, basting occasionally or until the chicken is browned and tender. Flame the chicken at the table by carefully pouring heated, flaming brandy over it. Serve immediately.

Yield: 12 servings
Exchange, 1 serving: 3½ medium-fat meat
Calories, 1 serving: 265
Carbohydrates, 1 serving: 1 g

Coq au Crème

Try this recipe—chicken with cream sauce.

2¼ lbs.	*frying chicken, segmented*	*1 kg*
	salt	
½ c.	*port*	*125 mL*
¾ c.	*skim evaporated milk*	*190 mL*
1	*egg yolk*	*1*
	fresh parsley, chopped	

In a nonstick skillet, slowly brown the chicken (you do not need any shortening); do not crowd the pan. Return all browned chicken pieces to the pan and add the wine and milk. Cover tightly and simmer gently for about 40 minutes or until chicken is tender. Remove chicken to a hot serving platter and place in a warm oven. Beat egg yolk and add a small amount of the wine mixture; stir to blend. Return to pan. Cook and stir over low heat just long enough to thicken the sauce. Pour over the chicken. Garnish with chopped parsley. Serve hot.

Yield: 8 servings
Exchange, 1 serving: 2½ medium-fat meat
¼ fruit
Calories, 1 serving: 200
Carbohydrates, 1 serving: 2 g

Arroz con Pollo

A colorful chicken entrée from Spain.

2¼ lbs.	*frying chicken, segmented*	*1 kg*
1 t.	*salt*	*5 mL*
¼ t.	*black pepper, freshly ground*	*1 mL*
1	*lemon, freshly squeezed*	*1*
2 T.	*olive oil*	*30 mL*
1	*onion, chopped*	*1*
1	*garlic clove, minced*	*1*
2 T.	*paprika*	*30 mL*
1	*bay leaf*	*1*
4	*whole cloves*	*4*
1	*fresh Italian oregano sprig*	*1*
3 c.	*boiling water*	*750 mL*
1½ c.	*long-grain rice*	*375 mL*
1 c.	*pimiento, sliced*	*250 mL*

| 6 | green olives, sliced | 6 |
| 1 c. | fresh peas, shelled | 250 mL |

Wash and season the chicken pieces with salt, pepper, and lemon juice; refrigerate for at least 5 hours or overnight. Pat chicken dry and brown in the oil in a nonstick skillet, turning frequently. Add the onion, garlic, paprika, bay leaf, cloves, and oregano. Pour into the skillet just enough of the boiling water to cover the chicken; cover and simmer slowly for 30 minutes. Stir in the remaining water and rice. Cover and cook an additional 10 minutes. Add the pimientos, olives, and peas; cover and simmer for 15 minutes or until all liquid has been absorbed.

Yield: 12 servings
Exchange, 1 serving: 2 lean meat
4 vegetable
½ fat
Calories, 1 serving: 234
Carbohydrates, 1 serving: 20 g

Mustard-Covered Chicken Breasts

The mustard flavor is sure to score praises from your guests.

4 (4 oz. each)	chicken breasts, deboned and skinned	4 (120 g each)
2 T.	Dijon-style mustard	30 mL
½ lb.	snow-capped mushrooms, sliced	225 g
1 c.	Chicken Stock	250 mL
1	parsley sprig, coarsely chopped	1

Using the bottom of a plate, press the chicken breasts until flattened. In a nonstick skillet, slowly and lightly brown each chicken breast on both sides; place in a lightly greased baking pan; do not overlap or stack the pieces. Spread the mustard over the chicken. Bake at 350 °F (175 °C) for 10 minutes. Top with the mushrooms and pour the stock into the pan. Sprinkle with the parsley, cover tightly, and return to the oven and bake 20 minutes more. Serve hot.

Yield: 4 servings
Exchange, 1 serving: 2 lean meat
Calories, 1 serving: 114
Carbohydrates, 1 serving: 2 g

Chicken Sauté, Mascotte

An Italian specialty from Mr. Mascotte.

4 (4 oz. each)	chicken breasts	4 (120 g each)
	salt, freshly ground pepper, and paprika	
2 T.	unsalted butter	30 mL
1 T.	fresh tarragon leaves	15 mL
1 T.	fresh rosemary leaves	15 mL
½ lb.	morels	225 g
1	lemon, freshly squeezed	1
½ c.	dry white wine	125 mL
2 T.	cream sherry	30 mL
1 T.	Chicken Stock	15 mL
6	small, cooked artichokes, halved	6
	fresh parsley, chopped	

Wash and season the chicken breasts with salt, pepper, and paprika. Using a large nonstick skillet, brown the chicken in butter, turning to brown all sides. Sprinkle with tarragon and rosemary leaves. Cover and cook over medium heat for 20 minutes or until tender. Remove breasts to 4 hot serving dishes and keep warm in a warm oven. Add the morels, lemon juice, wine, sherry, and stock to the skillet. Cook a few minutes; add the artichokes and heat until hot. Spoon vegetables over the chicken. Reduce the sauce over medium heat until smooth and thick; spoon over the warm chicken. Sprinkle with the parsley. Serve immediately.

Yield: 4 servings
Exchange, 1 serving: 3 medium-fat meat
1 vegetable
Calories, 1 serving: 246
Carbohydrates, 1 serving: 5 g

Pineapple Chicken, Hawaiian Style

4½ lbs.	roasting chicken	2 kg
	salt and freshly ground pepper	
1	bunch parsley	1
4	celery stalks with leaves	4
2 c.	fresh pineapple, cubed	500 mL
½ c.	sauterne	125 mL

Remove excess fat from the chicken; wash and dry the chicken and season with salt and pepper. Stuff the parsley and celery with leaves into the chicken cavity. Place chicken on a rack in a roasting pan. Bake at 350 °F (175 °C) for 35 minutes or until almost tender. Remove the parsley and celery from the cavity and spoon pineapple into cavity. Pour sauterne over the chicken; cover tightly. Return to oven and continue baking for 15 to 20 minutes more, basting occasionally. Add extra water to the pan, if needed.

Yield: 10 servings
Exchange, 1 serving: 4 lean meat
½ fruit
Calories, 1 serving: 247
Carbohydrates, 1 serving: 5 g

Glazed Chicken Breasts

The mixture of tart currant jelly and farmer cheese melts to form the glaze.

	PAM nonstick vegetable cooking spray	
4 (4 oz. each)	chicken breasts, skins removed	4 (120 g each)
1 t.	salt	5 mL
¼ t.	pepper, freshly ground	1 mL
½ c.	Red Currant Jelly	125 mL
¼ c.	Chicken Stock	60 mL
1 T.	lemon juice	15 mL
⅓ c.	farmer cheese, shredded	90 mL

Coat a nonstick skillet with the cooking spray. Over low heat, sauté the chicken breasts until lightly browned on both sides. (Do not crowd the skillet.) Sprinkle with salt and pepper. Combine the jelly, stock, and juice in a bowl or blender; beat until well blended. Pour over the chicken; cover, and reduce the heat. Simmer for 15 minutes; remove pan from heat. Sprinkle chicken with the cheese and place 5 to 6 in. (13 to 15 cm) from the broiler. Broil until cheese melts and the chicken top is slightly browned. Serve immediately.

Yield: 4 servings
Exchange, 1 serving: 2 lean meat
¹/₅ fruit
Calories, 1 serving: 165
Carbohydrates, 1 serving: 2 g

Roquefort and Herb-Coated Chicken in Tomato Sauce

A delightfully new flavor for chicken.

2¼ lbs.	roasting chicken	1 kg
1 c.	bread crumbs (made with fresh bread)	250 mL
1 oz.	Roquefort cheese	28 g
½ c.	fresh chive, chopped	125 mL
1 T.	fresh thyme, chopped	15 mL
1 t.	salt	5 mL
¼ t.	pepper, freshly ground	1 mL
1 c.	tomato juice	250 mL
½ c.	white onion, finely chopped	125 mL
2	tomatoes, chopped	2
	salt and freshly ground pepper to taste	

Wash and set the chicken on a roasting rack in 450 °F (230 °C) oven; roast for 20 minutes or until browned. Remove from oven and reduce the heat to 325 °F (165 °C). Combine the bread crumbs, cheese, chive, thyme, salt, and pepper in a food processor or blender; mix into a paste. (You can also do the mixing with your hands in a bowl; it just takes longer.) Press the mixture onto the chicken. Return to the oven and roast for 30 to 40 minutes or until chicken is tender. Remove chicken to a hot serving platter; keep warm. Combine the tomato juice, onion, and tomatoes in saucepan; cook for 5 minutes. Add remaining juices from the roasting pan; cook over low heat until the mixture is reduced and thickened to a sauce consistency. Spoon the sauce over the warm chicken or serve in a sauceboat.

Yield: 8 servings
Exchange, 1 serving: 2 lean meat
¼ bread
½ vegetable
Calories, 1 serving: 164
Carbohydrates, 1 serving: 7 g

Paprikahühner

A version of Austrian paprika chicken.

3 T.	unsalted butter	45 mL
2 c.	onions, chopped	500 mL
2¼ lbs.	frying chicken, cut in 8 pieces	1 kg
3 T.	all-purpose flour	45 mL

1 c.	Chicken Stock	250 mL
2 t.	salt	10 mL
2 t.	paprika	10 mL
1 c.	Dannon plain low-fat yogurt	250 mL

Melt the butter in a nonstick skillet; sauté the onions until tender. Lay the chicken on the onions. Cover and simmer over low heat for 45 minutes or until chicken is tender. Remove chicken to a hot serving platter; keep warm. Stir the flour into the onions in the skillet. Gradually add the stock and season with salt. Cook and stir over low heat until thickened; remove pan from heat. Stir in the paprika and yogurt. Return chicken to pan. Spoon sauce over chicken. Transfer to serving platter. Serve hot.

Yield: 8 servings
Exchange, 1 serving: 2 medium-fat meat
  1 vegetable
  ½ bread
Calories, 1 serving: 210
Carbohydrates, 1 serving: 8 g

Chicken, Sichuan (Szechwan) Style

4 (4 oz. each)	chicken breasts	4 (120 g each)
1 qt.	water	1 L
2 t.	salt	10 mL
½ t.	pepper, freshly ground	2 mL
⅓ c.	Oriental Sesame Sauce	90 mL
¼ c.	rice wine vinegar	60 mL
1 t.	chili powder	5 mL
1 t.	fresh ginger, finely chopped	5 mL
½ t.	garlic, finely chopped	2 mL

Remove bone and skin from the chicken breasts. Heat water and salt in a saucepan; when boiling, add the chicken and reduce the heat. Simmer for 30 minutes or until tender. Meanwhile, combine remaining ingredients in a bowl; stir to blend thoroughly. Remove chicken to a serving platter or individual serving dish. Spoon sauce over the chicken. Place under a broiler, 5 in. (13 cm) from the heat, for 5 minutes or until lightly browned. Serve immediately.

Yield: 4 servings
Exchange, 1 serving: 2 lean meat
Calories, 1 serving: ¾ fat
Carbohydrates, 1 serving: 2 g

Polynesian-Style Chicken

This is a favorite because it bakes in the oven and can be kept warm in case dinner is a little late.

4 (4 oz. each)	chicken breasts	4 (120 g each)
	salt, freshly ground pepper, and paprika	
2 T.	unsalted butter	30 mL
⅓ c.	pineapple-orange juice concentrate, undiluted	90 mL
2 t.	soy sauce	10 mL
½ t.	ginger root, freshly ground	2 mL
1	garlic clove, minced	1

Melt butter in a nonstick skillet and lightly brown the chicken breasts; place in a baking pan. Heat the concentrate, soy sauce, ginger, garlic, and ¼ c. (60 mL) water in a saucepan; pour over the chicken. Cover and bake at 350 °F (175 °C) for 20 to 25 minutes or until tender. Baste chicken occasionally, adding extra water to pan, if needed. If dinner is late, reduce oven heat to 200 °F (93 °C). Keep chicken well covered and baste occasionally.

Yield: 4 servings
Exchange, 1 serving: 2 lean meat
2 fruit
Calories, 1 serving: 203
Carbohydrates, 1 serving: 22 g

Enchiladas de Gallina

An exceptional recipe given to me by a Costa Rican native.

¼ c.	raisins	60 mL
½ c.	cooked chicken, finely chopped	125 mL
¼ c.	chive, finely chopped	60 mL
¼ c.	black olives, finely chopped	60 mL
12	tortillas	12
¼ c.	almond slivers, toasted	60 mL
2	eggs, slightly beaten	2
6	large tomatoes, chopped	6
½ c.	white onions, finely chopped	125 mL
2	chilies	2
	oil for deep-frying	
	salt (optional)	
1	iceberg lettuce head, finely chopped	1
½ c.	radishes, finely chopped	125 mL

Plump the raisins by pouring boiling water over them; soak for 10 minutes. Drain raisins thoroughly; place in a paper towel and pat dry. In a bowl, combine the plumped raisins, chicken, chive, olives, and almond slivers. Dip tortillas into the beaten eggs. Spoon a small amount of the chicken mixture down the middle of each tortilla; roll up. Heat the oil in a deep fryer; place tortillas, seam side down, in the oil. Turn tortillas and fry until golden brown. Transfer to a hot platter with a slotted spoon; keep warm. In a small saucepan, combine the tomatoes, onions, and chilies. Cook and stir over medium heat to make a thick sauce. Season with salt, if needed. Spoon sauce over the enchiladas. Garnish each serving with the lettuce and radishes.

Yield: 12 servings
Exchange, 1 serving: ½ lean meat
1 vegetable
⅓ bread
Calories, 1 serving: 86
Carbohydrates, 1 serving: 11 g

Chicken and Oyster Entrée

1 lb.	*chicken breast, boned*	*500 g*
2 T.	*butter*	*30 mL*
⅓ c.	*dry sherry*	*90 mL*
12	*oysters*	12
½ c.	*oyster liquid*	*125 mL*
¼ c.	*fresh parsley, snipped*	*60 mL*
	salt and freshly ground pepper to taste	

Clean, remove skin, and cut the chicken breast into 6 pieces. Melt butter in a nonstick skillet. Sauté the chicken until brown on both sides. Reduce heat, add sherry, and simmer until tender. Transfer chicken to a heated plate; keep warm. Place the oysters in the skillet. Add the oyster liquid and enough water to cover the oysters. When the edges curl and are cooked through, return chicken to the skillet. Add the parsley and salt and pepper to taste and baste with the oyster sauce. Remove chicken and oysters to a serving dish or 6 shell dishes. Spoon any remaining sauce over the chicken and oysters. Serve hot.

Yield: 6 servings
Exchange, 1 serving: 2 medium-fat meat
Calories, 1 serving: 142
Carbohydrates, 1 serving: 3 g

Sweet Goose

4½ lb.	lean young goose	2 kg
2 t.	salt	10 mL
1	egg yolk	1
2 T.	all-purpose flour	30 mL
1	garlic clove, minced	1
2 t.	brown sugar replacement	10 mL
1 t.	marjoram	5 mL
1 t.	Tone's nutmeg	5 mL
	salt and freshly ground pepper	

Soak the goose in cold water for 2 to 3 hours. Pat dry with paper towels; rub with salt and allow to rest for an hour. Cut goose in half. Place in a large saucepan and cover completely with boiling water. Cover saucepan and simmer for 30 minutes; drain thoroughly. Recover with more boiling water and continue simmering for another hour. Remove from pan with a slotted spoon. Meanwhile, make a roux of the remaining ingredients, adding enough water to give it a pouring consistency. Season with salt and pepper to taste. Pour roux over the goose. Place under a broiler for 5 to 6 minutes or until bird is slightly browned. Or bake in a 350 °F (175 °C) oven for 15 minutes or until bird is slightly browned. Serve immediately.

Yield: 10 servings
Exchange, 1 serving: 3 medium-fat meat
Calories, 1 serving: 265
Carbohydrates, 1 serving: 1

Oriental Curried Chicken

1 lb.	frying chicken, boned	500 g
	PAM nonstick vegetable cooking spray	
1 t.	cornstarch	5 mL
4 T.	curry powder	60 mL
1	onion, cut in half-rings	1
½ c.	Chicken Stock	125 mL
1 t.	soy sauce	5 mL

Wash, remove skin, and cut chicken into 1-in. (2.5-cm) pieces. In a cup, blend cornstarch with 1 t. (5 mL) cold water. Coat a wok or nonstick skillet with the cooking spray. Over low heat, stir-fry curry powder and onions until pungent. Add the chicken and stir. Increase the heat to high, add the stock and soy sauce; stir and cook for 5 minutes. Stir in the cornstarch mixture; stir and cook until thickened. Serve immediately.

Yield: 4 servings
Exchange, 1 serving: 2½ lean meat
½ vegetable
Calories, 1 serving: 145
Carbohydrates, 1 serving: 3 g

Mou Goo Gai Peen

This Chinese chicken dish with mushrooms is a favorite with many people I know.

½ lb.	*chicken breast, boned*	240 g
6	*dried Chinese mushrooms*	6
1 c.	*Chinese cabbage*	250 mL
¼ c.	*bamboo shoots*	60 mL
5	*water chestnuts*	5
12	*snow peas*	12
2 t.	*cornstarch*	10 mL
2 T.	*vegetable oil*	30 mL
1 t.	*salt*	5 mL
½ t.	*fresh ginger, grated*	2 mL
½ c.	*Chicken Stock*	125 mL
1 T.	*dry sherry*	15 mL

Remove skin from the chicken breast; cut chicken into thin slices. Soak mushrooms in warm water for 15 minutes or until soft; slice into strips. Slice cabbage, bamboo shoots, and water chestnuts. Remove strings from snow peas, and if large, slice diagonally. Blend cornstarch with 2 t. (10 mL) cold water. Heat a wok; add half of the oil, the salt, and ginger. Cook for 3 seconds. Add the mushrooms, cabbage, bamboo shoots, and water chestnuts. Cook and stir-fry for 30 seconds. Add the stock, cover and cook for 2 minutes. Remove vegetables to serving dish and keep warm. Reheat pan and add remaining oil. Add chicken and sherry; stir and cook until chicken turns white (when stir-frying, chicken will turn from pink to white when cooked). Return cooked vegetables to wok. When mixture begins to boil, add the cornstarch mixture; stir and cook until the mixture thickens. Serve warm.

Yield: 4 servings
Exchange, 1 serving: 1½ medium-fat meat
½ vegetable
Calories, 1 serving: 125
Carbohydrates, 1 serving: 2 g

Orange-Pineapple Chicken

4½ lbs.	roasting chicken	2 kg
	salt	
2 c.	cooked brown rice	500 mL
half	yellow onion, chopped	half
1 c.	canned pineapple cubes with their juice	250 mL
1 c.	snow-capped mushrooms, sliced	250 mL
½ c.	mandarin oranges	125 mL
½ c.	celery, sliced	125 mL
2 T.	slivered almonds, toasted	30 mL

Clean the chicken of all fat; salt the back and neck cavities. In a large mixing bowl, combine the rice, onion, pineapple, mushrooms, oranges, celery, and half of the almonds. Work with your hands until completely mixed. Stuff into the chicken cavities; secure with poultry pins or toothpicks. Place chicken in a large roasting pan. Add ¼ c. (60 mL) water to bottom of the pan. Sprinkle chicken with remaining almonds. Cover and bake at 375 °F (190 °C) for 1 hour. Remove cover and continue baking for 1 to 1½ hours or until chicken is tender. Allow 10 minutes for the chicken to rest before carving.

Yield: 12 servings
Exchange, 1 serving: 2 medium-fat meat
½ bread
½ fruit
Calories, 1 serving: 209
Carbohydrates, 1 serving: 11 g

Raemono's Supreme Chicken

2	bacon slices	2
1 c.	celery with leaves, chopped	250 mL
3	garlic cloves	3
5	green onions with 3 in. (7.5 cm)	5
	of the green part, sliced	
2 c.	chicken breast, cooked and cut	500 mL
	into pieces	
½ c.	red Lambrusco wine	125 mL
2 T.	fresh oregano leaves, chopped, or	30 mL
	2 t. (10 mL) dried oregano	

Fry bacon in a skillet until crispy. Remove the bacon, add celery, garlic, and onions to the skillet. Sauté for 3 minutes. Add the chicken, Lambrusco, and oregano. Reduce the heat, stir, cover skillet, and simmer until liquid has evaporated, stirring occasionally. Serve on hot rice or pasta, garnished with spicy apple ring and/or a parsley sprig.

Yield: 4 servings
Exchange, 1 serving: 1 lean meat
Calories, 1 serving: 85
Carbohydrates, 1 serving: 4 g

Stuffed Turkey Thigh with Fruit Dressing

2 (6 oz. each)	turkey thighs, deboned	2 (180 g each)
1	small apple, cored and quartered	1
4	dried apricots	4
1 slice	white bread with crust removed	1 slice
½ c.	all-purpose flour	125 mL
½ t.	baking powder	2 mL
1 t.	salt	5 mL
½ c.	water	125 mL
	vegetable oil for frying	

Remove skin and slightly flatten the turkey thighs. Combine the apple, apricots, and bread in a blender. On high speed, blend to almost a paste; occasionally, stop the blending to push food down from sides of the container. Divide the fruit mixture in half. Form into 2 balls; place a ball on each half of the turkey thigh. Fold edges together to form a pocket; pin securely. Place in freezer until outside meat is firm. Combine the flour, baking powder, salt, and water in a small, narrow bowl; whip into a thin batter. Dip each thigh in batter to completely coat; shake off excess, and place again in the freezer. When slightly firm, fry in hot oil until browned on all sides. Place on a baking sheet; bake at 350 °F (175 °C) for 25 to 30 minutes. Carefully remove pins and cut thighs in half.

Yield: 4 servings
Exchange, 1 serving: 1¼ lean meat
1 bread
½ fruit
Calories, 1 serving: 163
Carbohydrates, 1 serving: 20 g

Fresh Turkey Breast with Pecan Sauce

1 lb.	turkey breast, deboned	500 g
	salt	
	poultry seasoning	
2 t.	vegetable oil	10 mL
¼ c.	pecans, coarsely chopped	60 mL
¾ c.	water	190 mL
2 t.	cornstarch	10 mL

Remove the skin from the turkey breast; place the turkey in a baking dish; sprinkle with salt and poultry seasoning. Bake, uncovered, at 350 °F (175 °C) for 30 minutes. Brush turkey with the oil; return to oven and bake 15 minutes longer. Meanwhile, toast the pecans in a small nonstick skillet until browned. Combine the water and cornstarch and blend thoroughly; pour over the pecans. Cook and stir until liquid is clear (mixture will be only slightly thickened). Pour sauce over the turkey. Return turkey to oven and bake 15 minutes longer, basting with the pecan sauce at least 3 to 4 times while baking. Remove turkey to a heated platter. Spoon all the pecan sauce over the turkey. Serve immediately.

Yield: 4 servings
Exchange, 1 serving: 4 lean meat
Calories, 1 serving: 215
Carbohydrates, 1 serving: negligible

Smoked Breast of Turkey with Apricot Glaze

3 lbs.	boneless smoked turkey breast	1⅓ kg
½ c.	apricot nectar	125 mL
½ c.	cold water	125 mL
2 t.	cornstarch	10 mL

Place turkey in a roasting pan. Add about 1 in. (2.5 cm) of water; cover tightly. Bake at 325 °F (165 °C) for 1½ hours. Meanwhile, combine the apricot nectar, water, and cornstarch in a saucepan or bowl; stir to blend. Cook and stir over medium heat or in the microwave until mixture is clear and slightly thickened. Remove turkey breast from oven; drain the liquid. Reduce oven heat to 300 °F (150 °C). Pour a third of the apricot mixture over the turkey breast. Return to the oven and bake for 15 minutes. Pour the remaining apricot mixture over the breast and bake 10 minutes longer. Serve hot.

Yield: 12 servings
Exchange, 1 serving: 3 lean meat
⅕ fruit
Calories, 1 serving: 145
Carbohydrates, 1 serving: 2 g

Stuffed Roast Duck

In this version, the duck is sweetened with raisins.

3 lbs.	*young duckling*	*1.50 kg*
2 c.	*water*	*500 mL*
1 c.	*raisins*	*250 mL*
1 c.	*long-grain rice*	*250 mL*
½ t.	*vegetable oil*	*2 mL*
½ t.	*rum extract*	*2 mL*
	salt and freshly ground pepper to taste	
	fresh parsley sprigs for garnish	

Remove all excess fat from the duck; be sure to check both tail and neck cavities. Wash the duck thoroughly under cold water. Combine water and raisins in a saucepan. Bring to the boil, reduce heat, and simmer for 5 minutes; remove from heat and allow to cool. Drain, reserving both the raisin water and raisins. Combine the raisin water, rice, oil, and rum extract in a medium saucepan; bring to the boil. Reduce heat, cover and simmer, until all water is absorbed, stirring occasionally. Remove from heat and add the raisins. Season the duck with salt and pepper, including the interior of the tail and neck cavities. Stuff duck with the rice mixture; secure with poultry pins or toothpicks. Place duck, breast side up, on a large heatproof platter or pan with a rack (the platter should have a well to catch the grease). Bake at 350 °F (175 °C) for 2 hours. Drain grease often as it collects on the tray or pan. To serve; place the duck on a heated serving platter and remove the pins. With a small fork, move some of the dressing down onto the tail end of the duck. Garnish with the parsley.

Yield: 12 servings
Exchange, 1 serving: 1 high-fat meat
1 bread
½ fruit
1 fat
Calories, 1 serving: 242
Carbohydrates, 1 serving: 21 g

Roast Stuffed Pheasant

4 lbs.	pheasant	2 kg
½ lb.	freshly ground pork	250 g
¾ t.	black pepper, freshly ground	3 mL
½ t.	ground sage	2 mL
¼ t.	Tone's ground thyme	1 mL
⅛ t.	celery seed	½ mL
dash of each	ground ginger, nutmeg, and cayenne pepper	dash of each
1	green apple, cored and chopped	1
⅓ c.	fresh parsley, finely snipped	90 mL
1	egg	1
½ c.	dry sherry	125 mL
1 T.	lemon juice, freshly squeezed	15 mL
	salt and freshly ground pepper	

Clean and prepare the pheasant for roasting. Combine the pork, black pepper, sage, thyme, celery seed, ginger, nutmeg, and cayenne pepper in a bowl. Stir or work with your hands until well blended. Add apple, parsley, and egg; mix thoroughly. Adjust the seasonings with salt and black pepper. Stuff mixture into the pheasant. Place pheasant on a rack in a shallow roasting pan and cover with an aluminum tent. Roast at 350 °F (175 °C) for an hour or until tender. Remove aluminum. Combine the sherry and lemon juice; pour over the pheasant. Return to the oven and continue baking for 15 minutes, basting with pan juices every 5 minutes.

Yield: 10 servings
Exchange, 1 serving: 4½ lean meat
⅕ fruit
Calories, 1 serving: 282
Carbohydrates, 1 serving: 2 g

Wild Pheasant

Grill the pheasant with white chablis-oil marinade.

1½ lbs.	wild pheasant, cut into serving pieces	750 g
¼ c.	white chablis	60 mL
¼ c.	vegetable oil	60 mL

Clean and prepare the pheasant for broiling. Prepare medium-hot coals; or preheat a gas barbecue to medium high. Pour chablis into a blender, cover, and whip on high speed. Slowly pour the oil through the feed tube; blend for 3 minutes to make the marinade. Brush a side of each piece of pheasant with the marinade; place the oiled side down. Brush top side of each piece. Continue cooking, turning, and basting for 30 to 40 minutes or until the pheasant is done. Serve hot.

Yield: 4 servings
Exchange, 1 serving: 3 medium-fat meat
1 fat
Calories, 1 serving: 267
Carbohydrates, 1 serving: negligible

Wild Pheasant in Plum Sauce

1½ lbs.	wild pheasant	750 g
¼ c.	cornstarch	60 mL
1 t.	salt	5 mL
1 c.	vegetable oil	250 mL
½ t.	black pepper, freshly ground	2 mL
1 lb.	dark purple plums, pitted	450 g
½ c.	granulated sugar replacement	125 mL
1	garlic clove	1
½ c.	water	125 mL

Clean and cut the pheasant into serving pieces. Place the cornstarch, salt, and pepper in a plastic bag. Add the pheasant, a piece at a time, to the bag; shake to coat the pheasant and shake to remove any excess cornstarch. Pour oil into an electric skillet. Heat oil to 350 °F (175 °C). Brown the coated pheasant pieces in the hot oil, turning often. When browned, place pheasant on a heated platter and keep warm. Discard remaining oil, but leave the meat drippings stuck to the bottom of the pan. Combine the plums, sugar replacement, garlic, and water in a blender; blend at high speed until puréed. Pour the plum liquid into the skillet. Scrape up the meat drippings into the plum mixture. Return the pheasant to the skillet. Spoon plum sauce over the pheasant pieces. Heat to the boiling point, reduce heat to 250 °F (120 °C) and cook for 45 to 50 minutes or until the pheasant is tender. Occasionally, turn pheasant and spoon sauce over the top.

Yield: 4 servings
Exchange, 1 serving: 3 medium-fat meat
2 fruit
1 fat
Calories, 1 serving: 347
Carbohydrates, 1 serving: 21 g

Fresh Quail with Port Wine Sauce

6	fresh quail	6
2	bacon slices	2
½ c.	green onions, finely chopped	125 mL
2	whole cloves	2
1 t.	peppercorns	5 mL
2	garlic cloves, finely chopped	2
1	small bay leaf	1
2 c.	port	500 mL
½ t.	salt	2 mL
¼ t.	black pepper, freshly ground	1 mL
2 t.	chive, snipped	10 mL
2 c.	skim evaporated milk	500 mL

Wash and dry the quail. Fry the bacon in a nonstick skillet until crisp; remove and reserve. Add the onion, cloves, peppercorns, garlic, and bay leaf; sauté for 2 minutes. Add the quail and brown on all sides. Add the port, salt, pepper, and chive. Cover, reduce heat and simmer for 30 minutes. Remove quail to a heated platter and keep hot. Strain the sauce; pour sauce into the skillet. Add the milk; cook and stir over medium heat until hot. Pour sauce over the quail. Serve hot.

Yield: 6 servings
Exchange, 1 serving: 4½ medium-fat meats
½ non fat milk
Calories, 1 serving: 379
Carbohydrates, 1 serving: 7 g

Partridge with Sweet-and-Sour Cherry Sauce

2	partridges, dressed and quartered	2
2 T.	vegetable oil	30 mL
1 recipe	Sweet-and-Sour Cherry Sauce	1 recipe
½ c.	water	125 mL
¼ c.	dry white wine	60 mL

Brown the partridges on all sides in hot oil in a nonstick skillet. Add the remaining ingredients. Bring to the boil, cover, reduce heat, and simmer about 35 to 45 minutes or until birds are tender. Add extra water, if the sauce becomes too thick. Occasionally spoon the sauce over the birds.

Yield: 4 servings
Exchange, 1 serving: 4½ medium-fat meat
½ fruit
Calories, 1 serving: 359
Carbohydrates, 1 serving: 5 g

Sauces

Many authorities consider the sauce the gourmet touch to any entrée. It is the sauce that tells your family and guests that you have lovingly prepared the meal down to the last and finest detail. Indeed, a sauce is an elegant added attraction at most dinners or dinner parties.

You can make marvelous sauces for meat, poultry, game, eggs, vegetables, and desserts as well as for leftovers. Some sauces are tart, others are sweet; some are brown, others are white. When you are deciding on a sauce, think of the color and flavor of the sauce as well as of the entrée.

Tartar Sauce

The flavor of this sauce ripens over a longer period of time. I like to make it at least a day in advance.

1 t.	onion, minced	5 mL
2 t.	sweet pickle, finely chopped	10 mL
2 t.	stuffed green olive, finely chopped	10 mL
2 t.	capers, minced	10 mL
1 T.	fresh parsley, minced	15 mL
1 c.	low-calorie mayonnaise	250 mL
1 T.	tarragon vinegar	15 mL

Combine the onion, pickle, olive, capers, and parsley in a small bowl. Press with the back of a spoon or your fist and completely drain excess liquid. Fold in the mayonnaise and vinegar. Chill at least 2 hours before using.

Yield: 1 c. (250 mL) or 16 servings
Exchange, 1 serving: ½ fat
Calories, 1 serving: 20
Carbohydrates, 1 serving: 2 g

White Sauce

Thin:

1 T.	low-calorie margarine	15 mL
1 T.	all-purpose flour	15 mL

Medium:

1 T.	low-calorie margarine	15 mL
2 T.	all-purpose flour	30 mL

Thick:

1 T.	low-calorie margarine	15 mL
3 T.	all-purpose flour	45 mL

Other ingredients for all white sauces:

1 c.	skim milk	250 mL
½ t.	salt	2 mL
¼ t.	pepper, freshly ground	1 mL

Melt the margarine in a saucepan. Stir in flour and mix until smooth. Slowly add milk. Cook and stir continually over moderate heat until the sauce boils and thickens to the desired consistency; remove from heat. Stir in the salt and pepper. Use as needed in various recipes.

Yield: 1 c. (250 mL) or 16 servings
Thin sauce:
Exchange, 1 serving: $1/_7$ bread
Calories, 1 serving: 10
Carbohydrates, 1 serving: 1 g
Medium sauce:
Exchange, 1 serving: $1/_7$ bread
Calories, 1 serving: 11
Carbohydrates, 1 serving: 1 g
Thick sauce:
Exchange, 1 serving: $1/_7$ bread
Calories, 1 serving: 13
Carbohydrates, 1 serving: 1½ g

Cocktail Sauce

Serve with shrimp, crabmeat, or clams.

½ c.	chili sauce	125 mL
½ c.	catsup	125 mL
2 T.	lemon juice, freshly squeezed	30 mL
1 T.	horseradish	15 mL

1 T.	Worcestershire sauce	15 mL
1 t.	Tabasco sauce	5 mL

Combine all ingredients in a blender; beat to blend well. Chill before using.

Yield: 1 ¼ c. (310 mL)
Exchange, ¼ c. (60 mL): 1 fruit
Calories, ¼ c. (60 mL): 46
Carbohydrates, ¼ c. (60 mL): 11 g

Teriyaki Marinade

⅓ c.	soy sauce	90 mL
2 T.	red wine vinegar	30 mL
2 T.	granulated sugar replacement	30 mL
2 t.	salt	10 mL
1 t.	ground ginger	5 mL
½ t.	garlic powder	2 mL

Blend all the ingredients well. This marinade may be used with any meat or game.

Yield: ½ c. (125 mL)
Exchange: negligible
Calories: negligible
Carbohydrates: 2 g

Mustard Sauce

A real favorite to serve with German dishes.

2 T.	Dijon-style mustard	30 mL
1 T.	fresh horseradish	15 mL
3 T.	sweet pickle relish	45 mL
2 T.	low-calorie mayonnaise	30 mL
2 T.	catsup	30 mL
¼ t.	Tabasco sauce	1 mL

Combine all ingredients in a blender or bowl; beat until smooth. Refrigerate until ready to use.

Yield: ½ c. (125 mL) or 8 servings
Exchange, 1 serving: ⅕ fruit
Calories, 1 serving: 7
Carbohydrates, 1 serving: 1 g

Dill Sauce

A nice accompaniment for fish, snails, or oysters.

2 c.	onions, finely chopped	500 mL
½ c.	water	125 mL
1 T.	low-calorie margarine	15 mL
1 T.	all-purpose flour	15 mL
1 c.	skim milk	250 mL
⅓ c.	dill pickle, finely chopped	90 mL
1 t.	fresh dillseed	5 mL
3 T.	fresh parsley, snipped	45 mL
	salt and freshly ground pepper to taste	

Combine the onion and water in a saucepan; simmer until onions are tender. Drain thoroughly. Melt margarine in another saucepan or small skillet; blend in the flour to make a smooth paste. Slowly add the milk, cooking and stirring until slightly thickened. Add the onions and remaining ingredients. Stir and heat just to the boiling point. Serve hot or cold.

Yield: 2½ c. (625 mL) or 40 servings
Exchange, 1 serving: ¼ vegetable
Calories, 1 serving: 7
Carbohydrates, 1 serving: 1 g

Sultana Wine Sauce

This sauce is really good on ham.

1¼ c.	champagne	310 mL
¼ c.	sultanas, finely chopped	60 mL
2 T.	fresh ham, minced	30 mL
2 t.	cornstarch	10 mL
1 T.	cold water	15 mL
1 t.	low-calorie margarine	5 mL

Combine the champagne, sultanas, and ham in a saucepan. Simmer for 8 minutes. Blend the cornstarch and water in a cup; slowly add to the champagne mixture. Cook and stir over low heat until mixture thickens. Remove from heat and stir in the margarine. Serve warm.

Yield: 10 servings
Exchange, 1 serving: 1 fruit
Calories, 1 serving: 23
Carbohydrates, 1 serving: 6 g

Barbecue Basting Sauce

This sauce gives lamb, chicken, or veal a light herby flavor even without adding an herb.

½ c.	lemon juice	125 mL
½ c.	red wine vinegar	125 mL
¼ c.	soy sauce	60 mL
¼ c.	vegetable oil	60 mL

Combine all ingredients in a blender or bowl; beat to blend. Pour into a storage jar to save. Refrigerate until ready to use. Shake just before using.

Yield: 1½ c. (375 mL)
Exchange, ¼ c. (60 mL): 2 fat
Calories, ¼ c. (60 mL): 80
Carbohydrates, ¼ c (60 mL): negligible

Gooseberry Sauce

Gooseberries are a little hard to find, but you may try growing a gooseberry bush or look around for someone who has one. This is a version of a recipe that was given to me by an Englishwoman I lived with while working in Canada.

2 c.	fresh gooseberries	500 mL
1 c.	water	250 mL
2 t.	unsalted butter	10 mL
¼ t.	grated nutmeg	1 mL
¼ t.	ground allspice	1 mL
2 env.	Equal low-calorie sweetener	2 env.

Combine the gooseberries and water in a saucepan; cook until berries are soft. Cool slightly. Spoon berries into a blender, including some of the liquid; beat to purée. Return to the pan but do not place back over the heat. Add the butter, nutmeg, and allspice and stir to blend thoroughly. When you can put your finger all the way down into the mixture or place your hand flat on the bottom of the pan, stir in the sweetener. Serve warm or cold.

Yield: 20 servings
Exchange, 1 serving: ⅕ fruit
Calories, 1 serving: 7
Carbohydrates, 1 serving: 1 g

Chateaubriand Sauce

1 c.	champagne	250 mL
1	shallot, chopped	1
2 t.	Diet Fleischmann's margarine	10 mL
3 T.	very concentrated meat stock	45 mL
1 t.	fresh tarragon leaves, minced	5 mL
¼ t.	lemon juice, freshly squeezed	1 mL

Sauté the champagne with the shallot in the margarine for 3 minutes. Add the remaining ingredients and cook until very hot. Pour into a heated serving dish or directly on hot meat.

Yield: ¾ c. (190 mL)
Exchange: 1 fruit
⅔ fat
Calories: 73
Carbohydrates: 9 g

Creole Sauce

I have been asked for this Creole Sauce recipe so many, many times. It is exceptionally easy and has a truly authentic flavor.

¼ c.	green pepper, finely chopped	60 mL
3 T.	white onion, chopped	45 mL
2 T.	low-calorie margarine	30 mL
1½ c.	tomatoes, peeled, seeded, and chopped	375 mL
10	snow-capped mushrooms, sliced thin	10
1 T.	parsley, finely snipped	15 mL
	salt and freshly ground pepper to taste	
1 T.	cream sherry	15 mL

Sauté the green pepper and onions in the margarine until onions are translucent. Add the tomatoes, mushrooms, and parsley; simmer over low heat for 15 minutes, stirring occasionally. Adjust seasoning to taste with salt and pepper. Remove from heat and add the sherry. Serve hot.

Yield: 2 c. (500 mL)
Exchange, ¼ c. (60 mL): 1 vegetable
Calories, ¼ c. (60 mL): 23
Carbohydrates, ¼ c. (60 mL): 3 g

Red Currant Jelly

3 qts.	fresh currants	3 L
1 c.	water	250 mL
1 T.	lemon juice, freshly squeezed	15 mL
3–4 drops	red food coloring	3–4 drops
½ c.	granulated sugar replacement	125 mL
1 pkg.	Slim Set jelling mix	1 pkg.

In a blender or food processor, crush the currants; pour into a large saucepan. Add the water and bring to the boil. Reduce heat, cover, and simmer for 15 minutes; cool slightly. Pour mixture into a jelly cloth or bag and squeeze out juice into a large saucepan. Add the lemon juice, food coloring, sugar replacement, and jelling mix; stir to completely dissolve. Place over high heat; bring to the boil and boil hard for 2 minutes, stirring constantly. Remove from heat, skim off any foam from the surface. Pour into jelly glasses, leaving ½ in. (1.25 cm) space at the top for sealing. Seal with hot paraffin or sealing lid.

Yield: 4 c. (1 L) or 30 servings
Exchange, 1 serving: ⅕ fruit
Calories, 1 serving: 8
Carbohydrates, 1 serving: 1 g

Sweet-and-Sour Cherry Sauce

⅔ c.	cherry juice (from tart cherries)	180 mL
⅓ c.	white vinegar	90 mL
⅓ c.	granulated sugar replacement	90 mL
2 T.	green pepper, chopped	30 mL
1 T.	lemon juice, freshly squeezed	15 mL
1 T.	cornstarch	15 mL
⅛ t.	Tone's ground ginger	½ mL
dash	garlic powder	dash

Combine all ingredients in a blender. Blend until the green pepper is puréed. Pour into a saucepan, cook, and stir over low heat until mixture is clear and slightly thickened. Use as directed in the recipe or refrigerate. This sauce may be reheated. If sauce becomes too thick, add a small amount of water, stir, and reheat. Serve hot or cold.

Yield: ¾ c. (190 mL) or 4 servings
Exchange, 1 serving: ½ fruit
Calories, 1 serving: 22
Carbohydrates, 1 serving: 5 g

Oriental Sesame Sauce

1 c.	water	250 mL
½ c.	sesame seeds, toasted and ground	125 mL
¼ c.	He-she-ko onions, finely chopped	60 mL
1	garlic clove, crushed	1
1 t.	salt	5 mL
1 t.	cornstarch	5 mL
½ t.	ground ginger	2 mL
dash	Tone's chili powder	dash

Combine water, sesame seeds, onions, garlic, and salt in a small saucepan. Bring to the boil, reduce heat, and simmer, covered, for 2 minutes; remove from heat. Pour into a blender. In a cup, mix the cornstarch with 1 T. (15 mL) cold water; add to the blender with the remaining ingredients. Blend until smooth and onions are puréed. Pour into a saucepan. Cook and stir over low heat until mixture has thickened slightly. Use as directed in the recipe.

Yield: ¾ c. (190 mL) or 12 servings
Exchange, 1 serving: ¾ fat
Calories, 1 serving: 38
Carbohydrates, 1 serving: 2 g

Parmesan Cheese Sauce

2 T.	low-calorie margarine	30 mL
3 T.	all-purpose flour	45 mL
1½ c.	skim milk	375 mL
½ c.	Parmesan cheese, grated	125 mL
	salt and freshly ground pepper to taste	

Melt margarine in a saucepan; blend in the flour and work into a paste. Slowly add the milk; cook and stir until thickened. Stir in the cheese and cook 3 minutes more. Season with salt and pepper to taste.

Yield: 1¾ c. (440 mL) or 14 servings
Exchange, 1 serving: ¼ bread
½ fat
Calories, 1 serving: 44
Carbohydrates, 1 serving: 2½ g

Egg-Lemon Sauce

1	egg	1
3	egg yolks	3
¼ c.	lemon juice, freshly squeezed	60 mL
½ t.	fresh lemon peel, grated	2 mL
1 c.	hot chicken stock	250 mL

In a food processor or bowl, beat egg and egg yolks until light. Gradually beat in lemon juice and peel. With a slow trickle, beat in hot chicken stock. Use as a sauce for fish, veal, lamb, or vegetables.

Yield: 1½ c. (375 mL) or 12 servings
Exchange, 1 serving: ½ fat
Calories, 1 serving: 22
Carbohydrates, 1 serving: negligible

Chinese-Style Marinade

½ c.	Chicken Stock	125 mL
¼ c.	soy sauce	60 mL
¼ c.	orange juice	60 mL
1 T.	cider vinegar	15 mL
¼ c.	tomato sauce	60 mL
2	garlic cloves, minced	2
1	bay leaf	1
½	cinnamon stick	½
½ t.	salt	2 mL
¼ t.	ground allspice	1 mL
¼ t.	celery seed	1 mL

Combine all ingredients in a saucepan. Heat to the boiling point and boil for 2 minutes; cool to room temperature. Remove bay leaf and cinnamon stick. Use as directed in the recipe or as a marinade for any meat.

Yield: 1 c. (250 mL)
Exchange: 4 fruit
Calories: 144
Carbohydrates: 32 g

Tangerine Sauce

A tangy sweet sauce for meats or desserts.

1	tangerine	1
1½ c.	water	375 mL
1 t.	cornstarch	5 mL
1 env.	Equal low-calorie sweetener	1 env.

With a fruit zester or vegetable peeler, remove the zest from the tangerine. Place zest and ½ c. (125 mL) of the water in a small saucepan. Bring to the boil, reduce heat, and simmer until zest is soft and water evaporates by half or more; remove from heat and add remaining water. Pour mixture into a blender and add the cornstarch; blend for 5 minutes or until zest is completely puréed. Return to the saucepan. Simmer over low heat until mixture is slightly thickened and liquid is reduced by half; remove from heat. When you can place your hand on the bottom of the pan, stir in the sweetener. Use as directed in the recipe or as desired.

Yield: ¾ c. (190 mL)
Exchange: negligible
Calories: negligible
Carbohydrates: negligible

Vegetables

It always amazes me when people tell me they don't like vegetables. I love them. A beautiful arrangement or mixture of vegetables on a table gives it both color and life. These crisp delicacies can be the major attraction on any dinner table.

But how often I have been served a glob of something gray called "peas" or "beans." Many times, vegetables are ignored completely at dinner parties and restaurants. Or vegetables are overcooked, tasteless, and lacking in any kind of distinguishing color. This is sad, because vegetable cookery need not be dull or tasteless.

Cook vegetables until they are barely tender. They do not always have to be boiled. Try sautéing, braising, or lightly microwaving them. Use interesting combinations of color, texture, and flavor. Try different seasonings: a light whisper of nutmeg on plain green beans; a small amount of chopped chive; thin slices of sweet red pepper with a plain bowl of cauliflower. Your choices are endless.

But remember, vegetables are delicate. Treat them with respect, and you will be eating some of the finest food imaginable.

Sweet Potato Chips

I like these chips with pork, veal, or poultry.

2	sweet potatoes	2
2 c.	cold water	500 mL
1 T.	lemon juice	15 mL

Wash and peel the sweet potatoes. Using the thin slicer on a food processor or a sharp knife, cut into thin, even slices. Combine the water and lemon juice in a bowl. Add the sweet potato slices (the lemon mixture will keep the slices from discoloring); cover with ice. Cool for at least an hour. Drain and pat dry with a terry towel. Fry in deep fat at 365 °F (184 °C) for about 3 or 4 minutes or until browned; drain. Sprinkle with salt or aspartame sweetener.

Yield: 4 servings
Exchange, 1 serving: 1 bread
Calories, 1 serving: 80
Carbohydrates, 1 serving: 18 g

Sherried Sweet Potatoes

4	sweet potatoes	4
2 T.	skim evaporated milk	30 mL
1 T.	Diet Fleischmann's margarine	15 mL
3 T.	cream sherry	45 mL
	salt and freshly ground pepper to taste	

Boil the sweet potatoes until tender. Peel and beat with an electric mixer. Add the remaining ingredients and beat until fluffy. Scoop into 6 individual, well-greased ramekins. Bake at 350 °F (175 °C) for 15 minutes or until lightly browned.

Yield: 6 servings
Exchange, 1 serving: 1⅓ bread
                    ⅓ low-fat milk
Calories, 1 serving: 159
Carbohydrates, 1 serving: 20 g

Roasted Potato Medallions

New potatoes sprinkled with fresh parsley are very tasty.

| 1 lb. | small new potatoes | 500 g |
| 2 T. | vegetable oil | 30 mL |

           salt and pepper to taste
3 T.   *fresh parsley, minced*   *45 mL*

Peel and trim the potatoes into small medallions. Heat the oil in a large
nonstick or heavy skillet. Place potato medallions in a single layer on
bottom of the pan. Sauté over high heat until potatoes are golden.
Transfer potatoes to a well-greased baking dish. Bake at 375 °F (190 °C)
for 15 minutes. Transfer potatoes to a heated serving dish. Season with
salt and pepper to taste and garnish with parsley. Serve hot.

Yield: 6 servings
Exchange, 1 serving: ¾ bread
                          ¾ fat
Calories, 1 serving: 86
Carbohydrates, 1 serving: 10 g

Potato Supreme

A potato dish that needs no gravy.

1¼ lbs.	*new potatoes*	*500 g*
½ c.	*onions, minced*	*125 mL*
2 T.	*unsalted butter*	*30 mL*
1	*large egg, well beaten*	*1*
½ c.	*skim milk*	*125 mL*
1 t.	*salt*	*5 mL*
½ t.	*white pepper, freshly ground*	*2 mL*

In a saucepan, cover the potatoes with water and bring to the boil; reduce heat, cover, and cook until potatoes are tender. Meanwhile, sauté
onions in the butter until golden brown. Drain potatoes and cool slightly
with cold water; peel. Rice potatoes through a potato ricer into a large
bowl. Stir remaining ingredients and onions into the riced potatoes.
Spoon mixture into a well-greased baking dish or divide evenly among
6 well-greased ramekins. Bake at 375 °F (190 °C) for about 40 minutes or
until well browned.

Yield: 6 servings
Exchange, 1 serving: 1 bread
                          1 fat
Calories, 1 serving: 116
Carbohydrates, 1 serving: 15 g

Artichokes a la Gerard

I don't know the origin of this dish, but the recipe was given to me in New Orleans.

1	lemon	1
6	large fresh artichokes	6
1 lb.	plum tomatoes	500 g
½ c.	dry white wine	125 mL
½ c.	Chicken Stock	125 mL
1	large white onion	1
2 T.	olive oil	30 mL
Bouquet Garni:		
2 T.	coriander seeds	30 mL
2 T.	peppercorns	30 mL
1 T.	thyme leaves	15 mL
5	fresh parsley sprigs	5
2	large bay leaves	2
2 t.	salt	10 mL
1 t.	black pepper, freshly ground	5 mL

Squeeze the lemon and add the juice to a bowl of cold water. Place or drop artichokes into acidulated water as you work; keep them in acidulated water until ready to use. Cut off and discard the stems of the artichokes. Break or snip off the bottom leaves close to the base. Remove several more layers in the same manner. Trim the tips and base, leaving a 1-in. (2.5-cm) base. Cut the base section into wedges. Cut off the top two-thirds of each artichoke. Purée the tomatoes in a blender or food processor. In a glass bowl, combine tomato purée, wine, and stock; stir to blend. Peel and cut the onion into large chunks. Add olive oil to a nonstick skillet and sauté onions until golden brown; shake pan often to cook onion evenly. Make a bouquet garni using the coriander, peppercorns, thyme, parsley, and bay leaves. Add the artichokes, tomato mixture, and bouquet garni to the onions; stir to blend and season with salt and pepper. Bring mixture to the boil; boil for 10 to 15 minutes or until most of the liquid evaporates and vegetables are tender; stir occasionally to prevent sticking. Just before serving, remove the bouquet garni.

Yield: 6 servings
Exchange, 1 serving: 2 vegetable
*　　　　　　　　　 1 fat*
Calories, 1 serving: 82
Carbohydrates, 1 serving: 9 g

Stuffed Tomatoes

You'll enjoy tomatoes stuffed with herbs.

4	tomatoes	4
1 T.	olive oil	15 mL
1 t.	Tone's ground basil	5 mL
1 t.	Tone's ground thyme	5 mL
2	dry bread slices, finely crumbled	2
2	garlic cloves, minced	2
¼ c.	fresh parsley, minced	60 mL
1 t.	salt	5 mL
½ t.	black pepper, freshly ground	2 mL

Halve, core, and remove seeds from the tomatoes; be careful not to squeeze the tomato shell. Invert tomatoes on a rack over a bowl and drain for 15 minutes; reserve the juice. Place tomatoes, cut side up, in a baking dish. Sprinkle with olive oil, basil, and thyme. Bake at 400 °F (200 °C) for 10 minutes. Meanwhile, combine the remaining ingredients in a bowl; mix with your hand or a spoon. Divide bread mixture among the tomatoe shells. Drizzle with a small amount of the reserved tomato juice. Return to oven and continue baking for 10 minutes. Serve hot.

Yield: 4 servings
Exchange, 1 serving: 1 vegetable
½ bread
¾ fat
Calories, 1 serving: 154
Carbohydrates, 1 serving: 17 g

Italian-Style Broccoli

2 c.	cooked broccoli florets	500 mL
1	garlic clove, minced	1
2 t.	olive oil	10 mL
dash	Tone's cayenne pepper	dash

Heat olive oil, garlic, and cayenne in a small saucepan; cook for 1 minute. Pour mixture over the cooked broccoli and flip to coat. Serve immediately.

Yield: 4 servings
Exchange, 1 serving: 1 vegetable
Calories, 1 serving: 20
Carbohydrates, 1 serving: 4 g

Broccoli Amandine

3 c.	broccoli florets and stems, cooked	750 mL
1 T.	butter	15 mL
⅓ c.	green onions, finely chopped	90 mL
¼ c.	slivered almonds	60 mL

Cook broccoli in a small amount of water until al dente. Melt butter in a skillet; add onions and almonds. Cook and shake until onions are tender and almonds are slightly toasted. Pour over broccoli; shake or flip to coat.

Yield: 6 servings
Exchange, 1 serving: 1 vegetable
1 fat
Calories, 1 serving: 65
Carbohydrates, 1 serving: 5 g

Braised Lettuce with Herb-Carrot Butter

4	firm Boston lettuce heads	4
3 T.	unsalted butter	45 mL
1	carrot, shredded	1
1	celery stalk, sliced	1
1	fresh parsley sprig	1
1	bay leaf	1
½ c.	Chicken Stock	125 mL

Place lettuce heads in boiling water and blanch for 3 minutes; remove and trim. Cut heads in half lengthwise; drain on a rack. Melt butter in a heavy or nonstick skillet; add the remaining ingredients, cover, and cook for a minute. To braise, add the lettuce halves, cut side down, and bring to the boiling point; reduce heat and simmer over low heat for 20 minutes or until lettuce is tender, adding extra water, if needed. Transfer to a heated serving dish with a slotted spoon. Serve warm.

Yield: 8 servings
Exchange, 1 serving: 1 fat
Calories, 1 serving: 43
Carbohydrates, 1 serving: 1 g

Asparagus Parmesan

1 lb.	fresh asparagus	500 g
3 T.	unsalted butter, clarified	45 mL
3 T.	Parmesan cheese	45 mL
2 t.	lemon juice	10 mL
	lemon wedges or cut rings and tomato curls	
	for garnish	

Clean and cut off tough stem ends of the asparagus. Place stalks in a steamer over rapidly boiling salted water. Cover and steam for 20 minutes or until al dente. Place hot asparagus on a heated serving plate. Pour butter over asparagus and sprinkle with the cheese and juice. Garnish with the lemon and tomato.

Yield: 5 servings
Exchange, 1 serving: ½ *vegetable*
1¾ *fat*
Calories, 1 serving: 88
Carbohydrates, 1 serving: 2 g

Fresh Green Beans

A tasty combination – green beans with rosemary and ginger butter.

1 lb.	fresh green beans	500 g
2 t.	fresh rosemary	10 mL
¼ t.	Tone's ground ginger	1 mL
1 T.	unsalted butter	15 mL
	salt and freshly ground pepper (optional)	

Clean and snip the ends from the green beans. Sprinkle beans with fresh rosemary; place in a steamer over boiling water. Steam for 6 to 7 minutes or until tender. Melt butter in a nonstick skillet; stir in the ginger. When tender, transfer beans from steamer to skillet; toss beans in the ginger butter until coated. Season with salt and pepper, if desired. Serve hot in a heated serving dish.

Yield: 6 servings
Exchange, 1 serving: 1 vegetable
⅓ *fat*
Calories, 1 serving: 37
Carbohydrates, 1 serving: 5 g

German-Style Red Cabbage

This cabbage version has a sweet-sour flavor with a hint of cinnamon.

2 qts.	red cabbage, shredded	2 L
1 c.	Chicken Stock, boiling	250 mL
1	apple, peeled, cored, and chopped	1
3 T.	red wine vinegar	45 mL
1 T.	granulated sugar replacement	15 mL
½ t.	salt	2 mL
1	cinnamon stick	1
1	whole clove	1

Combine cabbage and stock in a large saucepan. Cover and cook over medium heat for 45 minutes. Add remaining ingredients; stir to mix. Cover and cook for 30 minutes longer. Transfer cabbage to a heated serving dish. Remove cinnamon stick and clove. Serve hot.

Yield: 6 servings
Exchange, 1 serving: 1½ vegetable
Calories, 1 serving: 35
Carbohydrates, 1 serving: 8 g

Cabbage Provencal

This is an excellent vegetable by itself, but it also makes a very colorful central focus, surrounded by a number of other vegetables, such as braised mushrooms or a combination of broccoli and cauliflower.

half	red cabbage	half
½ c.	water	125 mL
1 t.	fresh rosemary leaves	5 mL
1 t.	salt	5 mL

Clean cabbage and remove core, but do not pull apart. Combine the water, rosemary, and salt in a saucepan. Slip the cabbage, cut side down, into the water. Cover the pan, bring to the boil, reduce heat, and simmer for 10 to 12 minutes or until cabbage is al dente. Transfer carefully to a heated serving plate with the rounded side up.

Yield: 4 servings
Exchange, 1 serving: ½ vegetable
Calories, 1 serving: 13
Carbohydrates, 1 serving: 3 g

Creamed Spinach

A great dish with a touch of garlic.

1 lb.	fresh spinach	500 g
2 T.	unsalted butter	30 mL
¼ c.	onion, chopped	60 mL
1	garlic clove, minced	1
2 T.	all-purpose flour	30 mL
½ c.	skim milk	125 mL
2 T.	low-calorie lemon yogurt	30 mL

Thoroughly wash and trim the spinach. Blanch spinach in boiling salted water for 2 minutes; drain. Squeeze out the excess water; chop spinach. Melt the butter in a nonstick or heavy saucepan. Add the onion and garlic and cook over low heat for 10 minutes. Stir in the flour to make a roux; cook and stir for 1 minute. Slowly add the milk. Cook until sauce thickens. Add the spinach and simmer until thoroughly heated. Stir in the yogurt. Season with salt and pepper, if desired.

Yield: 6 servings
Exchange, 1 serving: 1½ vegetable
Calories, 1 serving: 40
Carbohydrates, 1 serving: 7 g

Buttered Beets with Spicy Wine Sauce

6	beets	6
⅓ c.	dry red wine	90 mL
¼ t.	allspice	1 mL
¼ t.	horseradish	1 mL
1 T.	unsalted butter	15 mL
	parsley sprig for garnish	

Wash, scrub, pare, and thinly slice the beets. Place slices in a saucepan and add the remaining ingredients. Simmer over low heat for 20 to 25 minutes or until beets are al dente and the liquid has evaporated. Spoon into a heated serving dish. Garnish with the parsley. Serve hot.

Yield: 4 servings
Exchange, 1 serving: 1 vegetable
½ fat
Calories, 1 serving: 52
Carbohydrates, 1 serving: 7 g

Baked Creamed Potatoes

You may prepare this dish in one large casserole or in small ones.

4 c.	potato cubes	1 L
¾ c.	skim milk	190 mL
⅓ c.	low-fat cottage cheese	90 mL
¼ c.	low-fat yogurt	60 mL
½ t.	smooth-leaf parsley	2 mL
2 T.	all-purpose flour	30 mL
	salt and freshly ground pepper	

Place the potato cubes in a well-greased 1½-qt. (1½-L) baking dish; or divide among 8 small casseroles or ramekins. Combine the remaining ingredients in a mixing bowl; stir to blend thoroughly. Season with salt and pepper to taste; pour over the potato cubes; stir just to mix. Cover and bake at 375 °F (190 °C) for 30 minutes. Uncover and bake 15 minutes longer or until lightly browned on top.

Yield: 8 servings
Exchange, 1 serving: 1 bread
Calories, 1 serving: 65
Carbohydrates, 1 serving: 13 g

Pearl Onions and Asparagus Tips

A very attractive combination served in a light cream sauce.

1 t.	vegetable oil	5 mL
20	fresh asparagus tips	20
½ c.	skim milk	125 mL
1-lb. jar	Aunt Nellie's whole onions, drained	500-g jar
3 T.	cold water	45 mL
1 T.	all-purpose flour	15 mL
	salt and freshly ground pepper to taste	
1 T.	fresh parsley, snipped	15 mL
¼ t.	paprika	1 mL

Heat the oil in a saucepan. Add the asparagus tips and shake to coat with oil. Shake and cook until tips are slightly tender. Remove asparagus from pan. Add the milk and onions to the pan. Cook over low heat until onions are warm. Combine water and flour in a shaker or small bowl; shake or stir to blend completely. Pour flour mixture into milk and cook, stirring gently, until the mixture begins to thicken. Add the asparagus and salt and pepper to taste. Fold the mixture to blend the ingredients. Heat until mixture is thickened and vegetables are hot. Pour into a heated serving dish. Garnish with the parsley and paprika. Serve hot.

Yield: 4 servings
Exchange, 1 serving: 1½ vegetable
⅓ bread
Calories, 1 serving: 61
Carbohydrates, 1 serving: 10 g

Delicious Perception

A medley of green spinach, red peppers, and white sprouts.

1 slice	bacon	1 slice
½ lb.	fresh spinach, cleaned	250 g
½	sweet red pepper, peeled and cut in julienne slices	½
1 c.	bean sprouts	250 mL
	salt and pepper to taste	

In a nonstick skillet, fry the bacon until crisp. Remove bacon and crumble. Cut the spinach; add to the skillet. Place over medium heat and sauté spinach until limp. Add the red pepper and bean sprouts. Sauté until thoroughly heated. Spoon into a heated serving bowl and top with the bacon.

Yield: 4 servings
Exchange, 1 serving: ¾ vegetable
¼ fat
Calories, 1 serving: 29
Carbohydrates, 1 serving: 4 g

Sautéed Cauliflower

1	cauliflower	1
	salt	
2 T.	olive oil	30 mL
	black pepper, freshly ground	

Remove all cauliflower leaves. Wash the cauliflower with cold water but do not break into florets. Place cauliflower in a large glass bowl; completely cover with a saltwater mixture containing 1 t. (5 mL) salt for every 1 c. (250 mL) of water; soak for an hour. Drain and cut into florets. In a saucepan, cover florets with fresh water. Cook until cauliflower is al dente; do not overcook. Drain thoroughly. Heat olive oil in a skillet. Add drained florets, shake, and cook quickly, until slightly browned. Season with salt and pepper to taste.

Yield: 6 servings
Exchange, 1 serving: 1 vegetable
1 fat
Calories, 1 serving: 71
Carbohydrates, 1 serving: 6 g

Pasta and Rice

Serving a pasta or rice dish either as the entrée or as a side dish often adds a distinct quality to a dinner. There are many great pasta and rice dishes from which to choose, but whenever you cook them, remember— pasta and rice should be cooked only until tender or al dente, not gummy and sticky.

For pasta to reach the al dente stage, it is absolutely necessary to use a large pot with rapidly boiling water. Add salt, if using, before adding the pasta. As the pasta softens in the water, fold it over gently to separate the pieces and keep them from sticking together. Also, a small amount of oil can be added to the pot at the beginning to help keep the pasta from sticking. When pasta has reached the al dente stage, quickly drain and pour it onto a heated serving dish. If you are adding pasta to a casserole, drain *before* reaching the al dente stage.

Cooking rice also can be a little tricky. But try one of these two popular methods to make tender rice. One way is to use 2 c. (500 mL) salted water for every cup of rice. Have the water boiling rapidly and slowly add the rice; stir or shake the pot to immerse all the rice in the water. Cover and reduce the heat as low as possible. Cook for about 15 to 25 minutes or until rice is tender. Another method is to have 2 qts. (2 L) of rapidly boiling, salted water; add 1 c. (250 mL) rice, stirring just to separate the grains. Do not cover. After about 15 minutes, check for doneness. When tender, rinse rice with hot water and place in a warmed oven to dry out. If you want to use the rice in a casserole, rinse in cold water until rice is cool. At this point, it may be refrigerated.

Shells a la BethAnn

A macaroni dish inviting with a light sour cream sauce.

7-oz. pkg.	large shell macaroni	198-g pkg.
1 T.	low-calorie margarine	15 mL
⅓ c.	leeks with green, finely chopped	90 mL
¼ c.	fresh mushrooms, chopped	60 mL
¼ c.	sour cream	60 mL
1 T.	skim milk	15 mL
	salt, freshly ground pepper, and paprika	

Cook macaroni as directed on the package; drain. In a skillet, heat the margarine and sauté the leeks and mushrooms until tender; remove from heat. Stir in the sour cream and milk until well blended. Fold into the cooked pasta. Season with salt and pepper to taste. Turn into a heated serving dish. Sprinkle with paprika. Serve hot.

Yield: 6 servings
Exchange, 1 serving: 2 bread
Calories, 1 serving: 150
Carbohydrates, 1 serving: 26 g

Finnish-Style Macaroni

A pasta version with a touch of horseradish. This is lovely when served in a pretty heatproof glass serving dish, garnished lightly with paprika and/or fresh, snipped parsley.

1½ c.	elbow macaroni	375 mL
1 qt.	skim milk	1 L
1 T.	butter	15 mL
2 T.	fresh horseradish	30 mL
1 t.	salt	5 mL
2	eggs	2
	black pepper, freshly ground (optional)	

In the top of a double boiler over lightly boiling water, cook the macaroni in the milk until almost soft, stirring frequently. Stir in the butter, horseradish, and salt. Slightly beat the eggs; add a small amount of hot milk from the pan to the eggs; then stir the remaining egg mixture into the macaroni. Cook until thickened. If desired, adjust seasoning of horseradish, salt, and pepper.

Yield: 6 servings
Exchange, 1 serving: 1 bread
                        1 medium-fat meat
Calories, 1 serving: 143
Carbohydrates, 1 serving: 17 g

Linguine of Venus Exquirere

L.O.V.E. You cannot ask for more than that.

1 recipe	*Tomato Pasta*	*1 recipe*
½ lb.	*boneless and very lean sirloin steak*	*250 g*
½ c.	*leek with green, sliced*	*125 mL*
10-oz. pkg.	*frozen chopped spinach, thawed and drained*	*285-g pkg.*
2½ c.	*skim milk*	*625 mL*
2 T.	*all-purpose flour*	*30 mL*
¼ c.	*sharp cheddar cheese, shredded*	*60 mL*
1 t.	*ground Italian oregano*	*5 mL*
2 t.	*ground Italian parsley*	*10 mL*

Make the pasta dough recipe. Cut dough into linguine shapes; dry for 20 minutes. Cook in boiling salted water until al dente; drain and keep warm.

To make the sauce: Chop (do not grind) the sirloin steak. In a nonstick skillet, brown the steak pieces; remove and set aside. Add the leek and spinach to the skillet and sauté for 3 minutes; remove from heat. Blend ½ c. (125 mL) of the milk with the flour until smooth. In a medium saucepan, combine the remaining milk, cheese, oregano, parsley, and flour mixture. Stir and cook over medium-low heat until thickened slightly. Stir in the sirloin and vegetables; heat just to the boiling point. Season with salt and pepper to taste. To serve, either place linguine on heated plates and top with the sauce, or place linguine on a heated platter and top with the sauce. Serve immediately.

Yield: 8 servings
Exchange, 1 serving: 1½ bread
                        1 lean meat
                        1 vegetable
Calories, 1 serving: 236
Carbohydrates, 1 serving: 27 g

Manicotti with Tomato Sauce

Pasta pancakes:

1 c.	all-purpose flour	250 mL
1 c.	water	250 mL
½ t.	salt	2 mL
4	eggs	4
¼ t.	olive oil	1 mL

Filling:

2.2 lbs.	ricotta cheese	1 kg
3	eggs, slightly beaten	3
½ t.	ground Italian parsley	2 mL
¼ t.	black pepper, freshly ground	1 mL
5.5 oz.-pkg.	mozzarella cheese, cut in 12 thin strips	167-g pkg.

Sauce:

3 T.	Amore tomato paste	45 mL
¼ c.	red cooking wine	60 mL
2¾ c.	water	690 mL
1	garlic clove, minced	1
½ c.	chive, snipped	125 mL
1 t.	ground basil	5 mL
½ t.	ground rosemary	2 mL

To make the pasta, combine the flour, water, and salt in a blender; blend until smooth. Reduce the speed to LOW and add the eggs, one at a time, beating on LOW after each addition. Heat the oil in a 6-in. (15-cm) non-stick skillet. Spoon 3 T. (45 mL) of the batter into the skillet. Roll the pan to cover surface with batter. Cook over low heat until firm, but do not brown; remove from skillet. Continue until batter is used and pasta pancakes are cooked.

For the filling, combine the ricotta cheese, eggs, parsley, and pepper in a bowl; stir to blend. Place 2 T. (30 mL) of the filling and 1 strip of mozzarella cheese on each pasta pancake. Roll up and place, seam side down, in a large shallow baking dish.

To make the sauce, combine all ingredients in a saucepan; stir to blend. Bring to the boil, reduce heat, and simmer for 15 minutes. Pour over the stuffed pasta pancakes. Bake at 350 °F (175 °C) for 35 to 45 minutes.

Yield: 12 servings
Exchange, 1 serving: 1 bread
2 high-fat meat
Calories, 1 serving: 261
Carbohydrates, 1 serving: 17 g

Linguine with Rhine Wine

3 c.	cooked linguine, hot	750 mL
1 T.	butter	15 mL
¾ c.	skim milk	190 mL
½ c.	Rhine wine	125 mL
2 T.	all-purpose flour	30 mL
¼ c.	water	60 mL
4	large ripe olives, sliced	4

Keep the linguine hot while making the sauce. Melt the butter in a saucepan; add the milk and wine. Combine the flour and water in a shaker or bowl; blend well and add to the wine mixture. Stir and cook to the desired thickness. Fold into the hot linguine. Turn into a heated serving dish. Garnish with the olives.

Yield: 8 servings
Exchange, 1 serving: 1½ bread
Calories, 1 serving: 100
Carbohydrates, 1 serving: 18 g

Tomato Pasta

You may use a pasta maker, but this dough is slightly soft for electric pasta makers.

1¾ c.	all-purpose flour	440 mL
1 t.	salt	5 mL
2 T.	Amore tomato paste	30 mL
2	small eggs	2

Combine flour and salt in a sifter. Sift mixture into a medium bowl. Make a well in the middle of the mixture; add the tomato paste and eggs. Using a fork, stir slowly, gathering in the flour around the edges. When mixture becomes too stiff to stir, work or knead it with your hands into a smooth, stiff dough. Divide dough in half and roll into 2 balls. Place dough on a lightly floured surface. Roll until very thin. Turn the dough frequently from side to side, around and around. Roll up the dough tightly, jelly-roll style. With a sharp knife, cut into strips of the desired width; dry at room temperature for 30 to 40 minutes. When ready to serve, cook in boiling water until al dente.

Yield: 8 servings
Exchange, 1 serving: 1½ bread
Calories, 1 serving: 110
Carbohydrates, 1 serving: 19 g

Stuffed Cannelloni with Parmesan Cheese Sauce

Italian sausage, spinach, and chicken are in the stuffing.

1 recipe	Cannelloni Pancakes	1 recipe
1 recipe	Italian-Style Herb Sausage (recipe follows)	1 recipe
10-oz. pkg.	frozen chopped spinach, thawed	285-g pkg.
1 c.	cooked chicken, diced	250 mL
¼ c.	Romano cheese, grated	60 mL
¼ t.	ground thyme	1 mL
⅛ t.	black pepper, freshly ground	½ mL
1 recipe	Parmesan Cheese Sauce	1 recipe

Prepare the Cannelloni and Italian-Style Herb Sausage. Drain the spinach thoroughly. Combine the sausage, spinach, chicken, cheese, thyme, and pepper. Stir or work with your hands to blend completely. Spread stuffing on cannelloni pancake. Roll up and place in a large baking dish. Cover with the sauce. Broil for 5 minutes. Serve immediately.

Yield: 18 servings
Exchange, 1 serving: ¾ bread
¾ medium-fat meat
Calories, 1 serving: 114
Carbohydrates, 1 serving: 13 g

Italian-Style Herb Sausage

2 T.	red Italian wine	30 mL
¼ t.	aniseed	1 mL
¼ t.	caraway seed	1 mL
½ lb.	lean ground pork	250 g
½ t. of each	fresh basil, oregano, parsley, and celery leaves, chopped	2 mL of each
2 t.	fresh chive, chopped	10 mL
½ t.	ground paprika	2 mL
¼ t.	ground cayenne pepper	1 mL
¼ t.	cayenne pepper flakes	1 mL
½ t.	salt	2 mL

Pour the wine into a bowl. Crush the aniseed and caraway seed with a mortar and pestle; add to the wine with the remaining ingredients. Mix with a spoon or your hands until thoroughly blended. Wrap sausage in plastic wrap and refrigerate for several hours or overnight to allow herbs to permeate the meat. Pan-fry and use as directed in the recipe.

Yield: 2 servings
Exchange, 1 serving: ½ high-fat meat
Calories, 1 serving: 156
Carbohydrates, 1 serving: 3 g

Cannelloni Pancakes

1 T.	unsalted butter	15 mL
1 c.	skim milk	250 mL
2	eggs, beaten	2
½ c.	all-purpose flour	125 mL
1 t.	baking powder	5 mL
½ t.	salt	2 mL
	PAM nonstick vegetable cooking spray	

Heat the butter and milk in a saucepan until the butter melts; remove from heat. Add the remaining ingredients and beat until smooth. Drop by spoonfuls onto a hot, nonstick skillet that has been coated with the spray. Fry until browned on both sides. Cool and use as the recipe directs.

Yield: 18 cannelloni pancakes
Exchange, 1 pancake: ½ bread
Calories, 1 pancake: 32
Carbohydrates, 1 pancake: 7 g

Fettucine Alfredo

½ lb.	fettucine	250 g
2 T.	butter, chilled	30 mL
¾ c.	Parmesan cheese, freshly grated	190 mL
¼ t.	black pepper, freshly ground	1 mL

Cook fettucine as directed on the package; turn into a heated serving bowl. Cut butter into 4 pieces; add the butter, cheese, and pepper to the hot fettucine and fold quickly to coat them. Serve immediately.

Yield: 10 servings
Exchange, 1 serving: 1 bread
½ high-fat meat
Calories, 1 serving: 142
Carbohydrates, 1 serving: 16 g

Hospitality Pilaf

½ c.	brown rice	125 mL
½ c.	wild rice, cooked	125 mL
½ c.	bulgur	125 mL
2¼ c.	water	560 mL
½ t.	fresh fennel seeds	2 mL
1 T.	olive oil	15 mL
2	celery stalks with leaves, chopped	2
1	red pepper, diced	1
1	small white onion, chopped	1
1	garlic clove, minced	1
5	large snow-capped mushrooms, chopped	5
2 T.	pine nuts, toasted	30 mL
2 T.	fresh coriander (cilantro), chopped	30 mL
1 t.	chili powder	5 mL
½ t.	ground cumin	2 mL
	fresh parsley and carrot curls for garnish	

Combine the brown rice and bulgur in a large saucepan. Add the water and stir; bring to the boil, reduce heat, cover, and simmer for 30 minutes or until water is absorbed; set aside. Heat the olive oil in a nonstick skillet. Add the remaining ingredients and sauté until al dente. Stir the vegetable mixture into the rice. Transfer to a heated serving bowl and garnish with fresh parsley and carrot curls.

Yield: 8 servings
Exchange, 1 serving: 2 bread
Calories, 1 serving: 125
Carbohydrates, 1 serving: 27 g

Italian-Style Rice

1 c.	brown rice	250 mL
2	carrots, chopped	2
1 c.	celery, chopped	250 mL
5	green onions, sliced	5
1	red onion, chopped	1
½	green pepper, chopped	½
½	red pepper, chopped	½
¼ c.	parsley, snipped	60 mL
3 T.	tarragon vinegar	45 mL
1 T.	vegetable oil	15 mL
	salt and freshly ground pepper to taste	

Cook the rice as directed on the package. Add the remaining ingredients and stir to completely mix. Serve hot.

Yield: 8 servings
Exchange, 1 serving: 1 bread
⅓ fat
⅓ vegetable
Calories, 1 serving: 105
Carbohydrates, 1 serving: 19 g

Rice Balls

¾ c.	cooked rice	190 mL
1	egg, separated	1
¼ t.	garlic, minced	1 mL
¼ t.	salt	1 mL
2 T.	all-purpose flour	30 mL

Combine rice, egg yolk, garlic, and salt in a saucepan. Cook and stir until mixture is hot and completely blended; cool. Form into balls. Dip in flour and then in egg white. Fry in deep fat at 350 °F (175 °C) until crispy and golden brown. Drain on paper towels.

Yield: 2 servings
Exchange, 1 serving: 1 bread
½ medium-fat meat
Calories, 1 serving: 127
Carbohydrates, 1 serving: 18

Fennel Rice

1 c.	long-grain rice	250 mL
2 T.	vegetable oil	30 mL
¼ t.	fennel seed, crushed	1 mL
2 c.	Chicken Stock	500 mL

Sauté rice in the oil until opaque. Boil fennel seed in the stock for 2 minutes. Add the sautéed rice. Cover and cook for 15 to 20 minutes or until rice is tender (add extra water, if necessary).

Yield: 8 servings
Exchange, 1 serving: 1 bread
¾ fat
Calories, 1 serving: 113
Carbohydrates, 1 serving: 17 g

Saffron Rice

2 T.	low-calorie margarine	30 mL
1	white onion, minced	1
2 c.	long-grain rice	500 mL
½ c.	dry white wine	125 mL
4 c.	chicken broth	1 L
½ t.	saffron	2 mL
½ t.	white pepper	2 mL
	salt	

In a large nonstick skillet, melt the margarine. Add the onion and sauté until transparent. Add the rice and sauté, stirring constantly, for 3 minutes or until rice is just becoming transparent. Add the wine and cook for 3 minutes. Add the chicken broth ½ c. (125 mL) at a time. Cook, stirring constantly, until liquid is absorbed after each addition. With the last addition of broth, stir in the saffron, white pepper, and salt to taste. Continue cooking until all liquid is absorbed. Transfer to a heated serving bowl.

Yield: 12 servings
Exchange, 1 serving: 1½ bread
               ½ vegetable
Calories, 1 serving: 127
Carbohydrates, 1 serving: 26 g

Baked Bulgur Pilaf

2 c.	bulgur	500 mL
¼ c.	low-calorie margarine	60 mL
1	onion, chopped	1
1 qt.	Chicken Stock	1 L
	salt and freshly ground pepper to taste	

Wash the bulgur under warm water. Drain and place in a well-greased casserole. Melt the margarine in a nonstick skillet; sauté the onion until tender. Add onion, chicken stock, salt, and pepper to the bulgur and stir to mix. Cover casserole and bake at 350 °F (175 °C) for 25 minutes. Uncover and stir with a fork; cover again and continue baking for 20 minutes longer.

Yield: 10 servings
Exchange, 1 serving: 2 bread
Calories, 1 serving: 154
Carbohydrates, 1 serving: 29 g

Bread

Bread—the staff of life—is so important in our life and diet that songs, poems, and prayers are written about it. History has been changed by it and religions are based on it.

Bread has changed a great deal from its early forms of unleavened morsels to today's light, fluffy loaves. In my home and many others, a meal is never complete without some form of bread on the table.

Spicy Muffins

1¾ c.	all-purpose flour	440 mL
1 T.	baking powder	15 mL
1 T.	granulated sugar replacement	15 mL
1 t.	salt	5 mL
2 t.	ground cinnamon	10 mL
1 t.	ground nutmeg	5 mL
½ t.	ground ginger	2 mL
2	eggs, slightly beaten	2
2 t.	vegetable oil	10 mL

Combine the flour and baking powder in a sifter; sift into a medium bowl. Add the sugar replacement, salt, cinnamon, nutmeg, and ginger; stir to blend. Add the eggs, oil, and just enough water to moisten; stir just enough to moisten dry ingredients. Spoon into 12 well-greased muffin pans. Bake at 375 °F (190 °C) for 20 to 25 minutes or until muffins test done with a toothpick.

Yield: 12 muffins
Exchange, 1 muffin: 1 bread
Calories, 1 muffin: 86
Carbohydrates, 1 muffin: 12 g

Raisin Muffins

1 c.	all-purpose flour	250 mL
1½ t.	baking powder	7 mL
dash	salt	dash
½ c.	boiling water	125 mL
¼ c.	raisins, chopped	60 mL
dash	ground nutmeg	dash

Combine flour, baking powder, and salt in a sifter; sift into a medium bowl. Pour boiling water over raisins; rest until cool. Add to the flour mixture with the remaining ingredients. Stir just enough to moisten. Spoon into 20 well-greased petite nonstick muffins pans. Bake at 400 °F (200 °C) for 20 to 25 minutes or until lightly browned. Turn out on a rack to cool or serve hot or cold.

Yield: 20 petite muffins
Exchange, 1 muffin: ½ bread
Calories, 1 muffin: 34
Carbohydrates, 1 muffin: 7 g

Pastry Shells

1	egg	1
dash	salt	dash
½ c.	skim milk	125 mL
½ c.	all-purpose flour	125 mL
	oil for deep-fat frying	

Combine the egg and salt in a bowl; beat to blend thoroughly. Add the milk and flour, beating just enough to blend. Heat a rosette cup iron in deep oil heated to 365 °F (184 °C); shake off any excess oil. Dip iron into the batter to within ¼ in. (6 mm) of the top. Dip again and cover completely with hot oil; fry until golden brown. Drain on paper towels. Cool on racks. Store in freezer or in a tightly covered container.

Yield: 10 shells
Exchange, 1 shell: ⅓ bread
Calories, 1 shell: 34
Carbohydrates, 1 shell: 4 g

Cranberry Muffins

1 c.	all-purpose flour, sifted	250 mL
2 t.	baking powder	10 mL
⅓ c.	cranberries, ground to mush	90 mL
3 T.	granulated sugar replacement	45 mL
¼ c.	low-calorie plain yogurt	60 mL
¼ c.	water, warmed	60 mL
⅛ t.	ground cardamon	.5 mL

Combine the flour, baking powder, cranberry mush, sugar replacement, and yogurt in a medium bowl; stir to mix. Add the water and cardamon; stir just enough to moisten dry ingredients. Spoon into 20 well-greased nonstick muffin pans. Bake at 400 °F (200 °C) for 20 minutes. Turn out on a rack to cool or serve immediately.

Yield: 20 muffins
Exchange, 1 muffin: ⅓ bread
Calories, 1 muffin: 31
Carbohydrates, 1 muffin: 5 g

Golden Nuggets

1 c.	all-purpose flour, sifted	250 mL
1 c.	water	250 mL
dash	salt	dash
1 t.	vegetable oil	5 mL
2	eggs, slightly beaten	2

Combine the flour, water, and salt in a bowl. Using a wire whisk, beat into a smooth batter; beat in the eggs. Lightly coat petite nonstick muffin pans with the oil; fill pans half full. Bake at 400 °F (200 °C) for 30 minutes or until golden brown and crisp.

Yield: 36 nuggets
Exchange, 2 nuggets: ⅓ bread
Calories, 2 nuggets: 26
Carbohydrates, 2 nuggets: 5 g

Flaky Scones

3 c.	all-purpose flour	750 mL
2 t.	baking powder	10 mL
¼ c.	unsalted butter, chilled	60 mL
1 c.	skim milk	250 mL
1	egg	1

Combine the flour and baking powder in a sifter; sift into a large bowl. Cut butter into small pieces and add to the flour mixture. Work with a pastry blender, forks, or your fingers until mixture is fine crumbs. With a fork, blend the milk and egg; remove 1 T. (15 mL) of the milk mixture from bowl and set aside. Pour remaining milk mixture into the flour; work into a dough (dough will not be smooth). Turn out onto a lightly floured surface; knead until the dough holds its shape. Place dough on a large baking sheet or jelly roll pan. Roll out the dough into a rectangle, 8×10 in. (20×25 cm). Without cutting through the dough, score dough into 1-in. (2.5-cm) squares. Brush dough with the reserved milk mixture. Bake at 350 °F (175 °C) for 25 minutes or until lightly browned. Serve hot or cold.

Yield: 40 scones
Exchange, 1 scone: ½ bread
Calories, 1 scone: 45
Carbohydrates, 1 scone: 7 g

Petite Pops

½ c.	all-purpose flour, sifted	125 mL
½ c.	skim milk	125 mL
dash	salt	dash
1	egg, slightly beaten	1
	PAM nonstick vegetable cooking spray	

Preheat the oven to 425 °F (220 °C). Combine the flour, milk, and salt in a medium bowl. With a wire whisk, stir into a smooth batter. Whisk in the egg but do not overbeat. Coat petite nonstick muffin pans with the spray. Fill the pans half full. Place pans in the oven, reduce heat to 400 °F (200 °C) and bake for 20 minutes. Prick each pop (on the side or top) with a poultry pin or toothpick. Continue baking for 5 to 10 minutes longer or until pops are very brown and sound hollow when tapped.

Yield: 18 pops
Exchange, 1 pop: ¼ bread
Calories, 1 pop: 20
Carbohydrates, 1 pop: 3 g

Ham Biscuits

2 c.	all-purpose flour	500 mL
1 T.	baking powder	15 mL
⅓ c.	ground ham	90 mL
¾ c.	skim milk	190 mL

Combine flour and baking powder in a sifter; sift into a large bowl. Mix the ham and milk; stir to loosen ham particles into the milk. Pour into the flour, stirring just enough to blend. Divide dough into 15 balls; pat each ball into a patty. Place on a greased baking pan. Bake at 400 °F (200 °C) for 10 to 15 minutes or until brown. Serve hot.

Yield: 15 biscuits
Exchange, 1 biscuit: 1 bread
Calories, 1 biscuit: 84
Carbohydrates, 1 biscuit: 12 g

Corn Bread

Corn bread with a hint of spice.

1 c.	yellow cornmeal	250 mL
1 c.	all-purpose flour	250 mL
1 T.	baking powder	15 mL
1 t.	granulated sugar replacement	5 mL
½ t.	salt	2 mL
⅛ t.	ground allspice	.5 mL
⅛ t.	ground nutmeg	.5 mL
1 c.	skim milk, warmed	250 mL
1	egg	1
¼ c.	low-calorie margarine, melted	60 mL

Combine the cornmeal, flour, and baking powder in a sifter; sift into a large bowl. Add the sugar replacement, salt, allspice, and nutmeg. Combine the milk, egg, and margarine in a separate bowl; whisk to blend. Stir into the flour mixture until just moistened. Turn into a well-greased and floured 8-in. (20-cm)-square baking pan; smooth the top with a spatula. Bake at 425 °F (220 °C) for 25 minutes. Cool on a rack for 10 to 12 minutes before removing from pan. Serve hot or cold.

Yield: 16 servings
Exchange, 1 serving: 1 bread
Calories, 1 serving: 79
Carbohydrates, 1 serving: 11 g

Butter Bread Sticks

4 c.	all-purpose flour, sifted	1 L
2 t.	granulated sugar replacement	10 mL
1½ t.	salt	7 mL
1 pkg.	active dry yeast	1 pkg.
¼ c.	water, warmed	60 mL
½ c.	butter	125 mL
⅔ c.	skim milk, warmed	165 mL
1	egg	1
1 T.	water	15 mL

Combine the flour, sugar replacement, and salt in a sifter; sift into a large bowl and make a well in the flour. Combine the yeast with warm water; stir to blend. Melt the butter in the warm milk. Slightly beat egg and water; add to the milk mixture; stir to blend. When milk mixture cools, beat into the swollen yeast. Pour the combined liquids into the flour well; beat with a wooden spoon until dough leaves sides of the bowl. Cover dough and set in a warm place to rise. When almost doubled, turn out onto a lightly floured surface; knead lightly. Roll out until ½-in. (13-mm) thick. With a sharp knife, cut into ½-in. (13-mm) strips. Using your hands, roll into sticks; then cut into 6-in. (15-cm) lengths. Arrange the cut sticks on an ungreased baking pan. Cover and rest for 15 minutes. Bake at 350 °F (175 °C) for 25 to 35 minutes or until golden brown and crisp.

Note: For a change, make seed or herb bread sticks. Follow this recipe, but before baking, roll the sticks in toasted sesame, poppy, or caraway seeds, or in dried onion or garlic flakes that have been crushed.

Yield: 36 sticks
Exchange, 1 stick: 1 bread
Calories, 1 stick: 79
Carbohydrates, 1 stick: 10 g

Crepes

3	eggs	3
dash	salt	dash
2 T.	vegetable oil	30 mL
1¼ c.	all-purpose flour	310 mL
½ c.	evaporated skim milk	125 mL
1 c.	water	250 mL

Place eggs in a blender and whip to mix well. Add the remaining ingredients; whip to blend thoroughly. Rest the batter for an hour at room temperature before using. Cook in a crepe pan according to manufacturer's directions.

Yield: 36 crepes
Exchange, 1 crepe: ⅓ bread
⅕ fat
Calories, 1 crepe: 32
Carbohydrates, 1 crepe: 4 g

French Bread

1 pkg.	active dry yeast	1 pkg.
¼ c.	water, warmed	60 mL
1 T.	vegetable shortening	15 mL
2 t.	salt	10 mL
1 c.	water, boiling	250 mL
¾ c.	water, chilled	190 mL
6 c.	all-purpose flour	1 L
1	egg white, slightly beaten	1

Sprinkle yeast into the warm water, let stand for a few minutes; then stir until dissolved and set aside. Place shortening and salt in a large bowl. Pour boiling water over shortening. Stir until shortening melts. Add the chilled water and cool to room temperature. Add the swollen yeast. Gradually beat in 5 c. (1.25 L) of the flour. Turn out onto a floured board. Knead in the remaining flour until dough is smooth and elastic. Place dough in a greased bowl; turn once to coat both sides. Cover and allow to rise until doubled. Shape into 2 oblong loaves. Place on a greased baking sheet; brush with egg white and make 4 diagonal slashes on top. Allow to rise; brush lightly with remaining egg white. Bake at 425 °F (220 °C) for 30 minutes; reduce heat and bake at 350 °F (175 °C) for 20 minutes longer.

Yield: 2 loaves or 32 servings
Exchange, 1 serving: 1 bread
Calories, 1 serving: 91
Carbohydrates, 1 serving: 16 g

Buttermilk Buns

These buns have a touch of caraway.

1¼ c.	all-purpose flour	310 mL
1 pkg.	active dry yeast	1 pkg.
½ c.	buttermilk, warmed	125 mL
1 T.	vegetable oil	15 mL
½ t.	salt	2 mL
½ t.	granulated sugar replacement	2 mL
½ t.	caraway seed	2 mL

Dissolve the yeast in the warm buttermilk; rest for 5 minutes. Combine the remaining ingredients in a large bowl; stir to blend. Pour in the swollen yeast and stir to mix. Turn out onto a lightly floured board; knead dough until smooth and elastic. Place dough in an oiled bowl and turn once to coat both sides. Cover and rest in a warm place until doubled in size; punch down. With your hands, form into 4 large or 8 small buns. Place on a greased baking pan. Cover with a towel and rest until swollen. Bake at 375 °F (190 °C) for 25 to 30 minutes or until lightly browned.

Yield: 4 large or 8 small buns
Exchange, 1 large bun: 2 bread
Calories, 1 large bun: 182
Carbohydrates, 1 large bun: 29 g
Exchange, 1 small bun: 1 bread
Calories, 1 small bun: 90
Carbohydrates, 1 small bun: 14 g

Desserts

Regal Custard

2 T.	granulated sugar replacement	30 mL
3 c.	skim milk, heated	750 mL
8	egg yolks	8
1 t.	vanilla extract	5 mL
3 T.	cream of cocoa	45 mL
6	egg whites	6
3 T.	granulated sugar replacement	45 mL
½ t.	vanilla extract	2 mL

Add sugar replacement to the hot milk; stir to dissolve. Beat the yolks until frothy; gradually beat in the hot milk mixture. Add vanilla extract. Pour into a well-greased 1-qt. (2-L) baking dish. Bake at 350 °F (175 °C) for 35 to 45 minutes or until a knife inserted in the custard comes out clean; remove from oven. Pour cream of cocoa over the surface. To make a meringue, beat the egg whites until stiff; gradually beat in the sugar replacement and vanilla extract. Spread half the meringue over the custard. Decorate with the remaining meringue, pressing it through a pastry tube or by dropping it from a teaspoon. Return to the oven and bake for 12 to 15 minutes or until meringue is a delicate brown color.

Yield: 12 servings
Exchange, 1 serving: ⅓ bread
½ high-fat meat
Calories, 1 serving: 74
Carbohydrates, 1 serving: 6 g

Apples in Honey

3	red Delicious apples	3
¾ c.	water	190 mL
1 t.	honey	5 mL
1 in.	cinnamon stick	2.5 cm
3	whole cloves	3
1½ t.	vanilla extract	7 mL

Core apple, making sure all the seeds are removed. Cut five 1-in. (2.5-cm) slashes down from top of the cored edge. Repeat cuts from the bottom cored edge. Combine remaining ingredients in a saucepan large enough to hold the apples. Bring mixture to boil. Add the apples, top side down. Reduce heat, cover, and simmer for 15 minutes or until the apples are soft. Place each apple on a heated serving dish. Finish the cuts through the apple, forming a flower on the plate. Spoon remaining sauce over the apples. Serve hot.

Yield: 3 servings
Exchange, 1 serving: 2 fruit
Calories, 1 serving: 80
Carbohydrates, 1 serving: 20 g

Fraises au Kirsch

Strawberries are always colorful and especially tasty with kirsch.

½ c.	fresh strawberries	125 mL
3 T.	kirsch, chilled	45 mL
1 env.	Equal low-calorie sweetener	1 env.

Wash and hull the strawberries. Place in a dessert dish and refrigerate until chilled. To serve, pour chilled kirsch over the berries. Sprinkle with the sweetener.

Yield: 2 servings
Exchange, 1 serving: 1 fruit
Calories, 1 serving: 38
Carbohydrates, 1 serving: 9 g

Truffles

2	egg yolks	2
7-oz. box	no-sugar white frosting mix	200-g box
2 T.	cocoa	30 mL
1 T.	brandy flavoring	15 mL

Beat the egg yolks until light and slightly thick. Add frosting mix, cocoa, and brandy flavoring; stir to blend completely. If needed, add water to make a workable paste. Shape dough into small balls. Place on waxed paper and refrigerate for several hours until firm. These truffles can be frozen.

Yield: 36 pieces
Exchange, 1 piece: ¹/₅ *bread*
        ¹/₂ *fat*
Calories, 1 piece: 38
Carbohydrates, 1 piece: 3 g

Blueberry Pudding

2 c.	all-purpose flour	500 mL
4 t.	baking powder	20 mL
½ t.	salt	2 mL
¼ c.	butter	60 mL
1 c.	skim milk	250 mL
1 c.	blueberries	250 mL

Mix and sift the dry ingredients. Cut in the butter. Add the milk and mix thoroughly. Fold in the blueberries. Pour into a greased pudding mould. Cover and steam for 2 hours or until done. Serve hot or cold.

Yield: 20 servings
Exchange, 1 serving: 1 bread
Calories, 1 serving: 76
Carbohydrates, 1 serving: 11 g

A Note on Products

The following manufacturers have given their permission to use their products in the recipes I developed for this book. For further information, write to the following addresses:

American Home Products
  Corporation
685 Third Avenue
New York NY 10017
Pam® nonstick vegetable cooking spray is a registered trademark of American Home Products Corporation.

Beatrice Grocery Products Division
P.O. Box 67
Clyman WI 53016
Produces Aunt Nellie's® products used in this book.

Brilliant Seafood, Inc.
315 Northern Avenue
Boston MA 02210
Produces shrimp products used in these recipes.

The Dannon Company
22-11 38th Avenue
Long Island City NY 11101
Manufactures Dannon® plain low-fat yogurt used in these recipes.

MCP Foods, Inc.
Box 3533
Anaheim CA 92803
Produces Slim Set® jelling mix for use in making jams and jellies.

Nabisco Brands, Inc.
River Road
East Hanover NJ 07936
Produces Diet Fleischmann's® margarine featured in these recipes.

Equal Consumer Affairs
NutraSweet Consumer Products, Inc.
P.O. Box 8517
Chicago IL 60686
Makes Equal® low-calorie sweetener used in these recipes.

Tone's
P.O. Box AA
Des Moines, IA 50301
Tone's®, the registered trademark for a full line of herbs and spices, has a salt exchange line where you can call a home economist to answer your questions: 1(800) 247-7517 (national) or 1(800) 372-6071 (Iowa).

Universal Foods Corporation
66 Broad Street
Carlstadt NJ 07072
Liberty/Ramsey Division produces Amore® brands used in this book.

Food Exchange Lists

If variety is the spice of life, Exchange Lists are just what you're looking for.

What do we mean by Exchange Lists? When we think of an "exchange" we automatically think of a "substitute" or a "trade." (I'll trade you an apple for an orange.) Basically, that's how it works, but the possibilities are endless.

Diets are sometimes stated in very dull, specific terms. For example:

Orange juice	1/2 cup
Oatmeal	1/2 cup
Rye toast	1 slice
Soft cooked egg	1
Butter	1 teaspoon
Milk	1/2 pint

Exchange Lists take the dreariness out of diets. The Lists are groups of measured foods of the same value that can be substituted in Meal Plans. Foods have been divided into six groups, or Exchanges. For example, vegetables are listed in one group and fats are listed in another group. Foods in any *one group* can be substituted or exchanged with other foods in the *same group.*

Within each group an Exchange is approximately equal in calories and in the amount of carbohydrate, protein and fat. In addition, each Exchange contains similar minerals and vitamins.

The number of calories in any food expresses the energy value of the food. As an adult you may need fewer calories to maintain normal weight. Many people as they reach their 30's and 40's become physically less active but do not change their eating habits. They store their excess calories as fat. The result: the famous "middle age spread." Your diet counselor will know how many calories you require each day to maintain good health.

Fats, carbohydrates and proteins are the three major energy sources in foods. The most common carbohydrates are sugars and starches. Proteins yield energy and contain nitrogen, which is essential for life. Fats provide energy and are the most concentrated source of calories. Alcohol also contributes calories.

Minerals and vitamins are substances present in food in small amounts and perform essential functions in the body. The foods of each Exchange make a specific nutritional contribution. No one Exchange group can supply all the nutrients needed for a well-balanced diet. It takes all six of them working together as a team to supply your nutritional needs for good health.

The exchange lists are based on material in the *Exchange Lists for Meal Planning* prepared by Committees of the American Diabetes Association, Inc. and the American Dietetic Association in cooperation with the National Institute of Arthritis, Metabolism, and Digestive Diseases and the National Heart and Lung Institutes of Health, Public Health Service, U.S. Department of Health and Human Services.

147

LIST 1 Milk Exchanges
(Includes Non-Fat Low-Fat and Whole Milk)

One Exchange of Milk contains 12 grams of carbohydrate, 8 grams of protein, a trace of fat and 80 calories.

Milk is a basic food for your Meal Plan for very good reasons. Milk is the leading source of calcium. It is a good source of phosphorus, protein, some of the B-complex vitamins, including folacin and vitamin B_{12}, and vitamins A and D. Magnesium is also found in milk.

Since it is a basic ingredient in many recipes you will not find it difficult to include milk in your Meal Plan. Milk can be used not only to drink but can be added to cereal, coffee, tea and other foods.

This List shows the kinds and amounts of milk or milk products to use for one Milk Exchange. Those which appear in **bold type** are **non-fat**. Low-Fat and Whole Milk contain saturated fat.

Non-Fat Fortified Milk

Skim or non-fat milk	1 cup
Powdered (non-fat dry, before adding liquid)	1/3 cup
Canned, evaporated—skim milk	1/2 cup
Buttermilk made from skim milk	1 cup
Yogurt made from skim milk (plain, unflavored)	1 cup

Low-Fat Fortified Milk

1% fat fortified milk (omit 1/2 Fat Exchange)	1 cup
2% fat fortified milk (omit 1 Fat Exchange)	1 cup
Yogurt made from 2% fortified milk (plain, unflavored) (omit 1 Fat Exchange)	1 cup

Whole Milk (Omit 2 Fat Exchanges)

Whole milk	1 cup
Canned, evaporated whole milk	1/2 cup
Buttermilk made from whole milk	1 cup
Yogurt made from whole milk (plain, unflavored)	1 cup

LIST 2 Vegetable Exchanges

One Exchange of Vegetables contains about 5 grams of carbohydrate, 2 grams of protein and 25 calories.

The generous use of many vegetables, served either alone or in other foods such as casseroles, soups or salads, contributes to sound health and vitality.

Dark green and deep yellow vegetables are among the leading sources of vitamin A. Many of the vegetables in this group are notable sources of vitamin C — asparagus, broccoli, brussels sprouts, cabbage, cauliflower, collards, kale, dandelion, mustard and turnip greens, spinach, rutabagas, to tomatoes and turnips. A number, including broccoli, brussels sprouts, beet greens, chard and tomato juice, are particularly good sources of potassium. High folacin values are found in asparagus, beets, broccoli, brussels sprouts, cauliflower, collards, kale and lettuce. Moderate amounts of vitamin B_6 are supplied by broccoli, brussels sprouts, cauliflower, collards, spinach, sauerkraut and tomatoes and tomato juice. Fiber is present in all vegetables.

Whether you serve them cooked or raw, wash all vegetables even though they look clean. If fat is added in the preparation, omit the equivalent number of Fat Exchanges. The average amount of fat contained in a Vegetable Exchange that is cooked with fat meat or other fats is one Fat Exchange.

This List shows the kinds of **vegetables** to use for one Vegetable Exchange. One Exchange is ½ cup.

Asparagus	Greens:
Bean Sprouts	Mustard
Beets	Spinach
Broccoli	Turnip
Brussels Sprouts	Mushrooms
Cabbage	Okra
Carrots	Onions
Cauliflower	Rhubarb
Celery	Rutabaga
Eggplant	Sauerkraut
Green Pepper	String Beans, green or yellow
Greens:	Summer Squash
Beet	Tomatoes
Chards	Tomato Juice
Collards	Turnips
Dandelion	Vegetable Juice Cocktail
Kale	Zucchini

The following **raw vegetables** may be used as desired:

Chicory	Lettuce
Chinese Cabbage	Parsley
Cucumbers	Pickles, Dill
Endive	Radishes
Escarole	Watercress

Starchy Vegetables are found in the Bread Exchange List.

LIST 3   **Fruit Exchanges**

One Exchange of Fruit contains 10 grams of carbohydrate and 40 calories.

Everyone likes to buy fresh fruits when they are in the height of their season. But you can also buy fresh fruits and can or freeze them for off-season use. For variety serve fruit as a salad or in combination with other foods for dessert.

Fruits are valuable for vitamins, minerals and fiber. Vitamin C is abundant in citrus fruits and fruit juices and is found in raspberries, strawberries, mangoes, cantaloupes, honeydews and papayas. The better sources of vitamin A among these fruits include fresh or dried apricots, mangoes, cantaloupes, nectarines, yellow peaches and persimmons. Oranges, orange juice and cantaloupe provide more folacin than most of the other fruits in this listing. Many fruits are a valuable source of potassium, especially apricots, bananas, several of the berries, grapefruit, grapefruit juice, mangoes, cantaloupes, honeydews, nectarines, oranges, orange juice and peaches.

Fruit may be used fresh, dried, canned or frozen, cooked or raw, as long as no sugar is added.

This List shows the kinds and amounts of **fruits** to use for one Fruit Exchange.

Apple	1 small	Apricots, fresh	2 medium
Apple Juice	1/3 cup	Apricots, dried	4 halves
Applesauce (unsweetened)	1/2 cup	Banana	1/2 small

Berries			**Honeydew**	1/8 medium	
Blackberries	1/2 cup		**Watermelon**	1 cup	
Blueberries	1/2 cup		**Nectarine**	1 small	
Raspberries	1/2 cup		**Orange**	1 small	
Strawberries	3/4 cup		**Orange Juice**	1/2 cup	
Cherries	10 large		**Papaya**	3/4 cup	
Cider	1/3 cup		**Peach**	1 medium	
Dates	2		**Pear**	1 small	
Figs, fresh	1		**Persimmon, native**	1 medium	
Figs, dried	1		**Pineapple**	1/2 cup	
Grapefruit	1/2		**Pineapple Juice**	1/3 cup	
Grapefruit Juice	1/2 cup		**Plums**	2 medium	
Grapes	12		**Prunes**	2 medium	
Grape Juice	1/4 cup		**Prune Juice**	1/4 cup	
Mango	1/2 small		**Raisins**	2 tablespoons	
Melon			**Tangerine**	1 medium	
Cantaloupe	1/4 small				

Cranberries may be used as desired if no sugar is added.

LIST 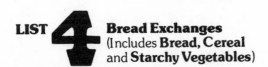 Bread Exchanges (Includes **Bread, Cereal** and **Starchy Vegetables**)

One Exchange of Bread contains 15 grams of carbohydrate, 2 grams of protein and 70 calories.

In this List, whole-grain and enriched breads and cereals, germ and bran products and dried beans and peas are good sources of iron and among the better sources of thiamin. The whole-grain, bran and germ products have more fiber than products made from refined flours. Dried beans and peas are also good sources of fiber. Wheat germ, bran,dried beans, potatoes, lima beans, parsnips, pumpkin and winter squash are particularly good sources of potassium. The better sources of folacin in this listing include whole-wheat bread, wheat germ, dried beans, corn, lima beans, parsnips, green peas, pumpkin and sweet potato.

Starchy vegetables are included in this List, because they contain the same amount of carbohydrate and protein as one slice of bread.

This List shows the kinds and amounts of **Breads, Cereals, Starchy Vegetables** and Prepared Foods to use for one Bread Exchange. Those which appear in **bold type** are **low-fat**.

Bread

White (including French and Italian)	1 slice
Whole Wheat	1 slice
Rye or Pumpernickel	1 slice
Raisin	1 slice
Bagel, small	1/2
English Muffin, small	1/2
Plain Roll, bread	1
Frankfurter Roll	1/2
Hamburger Bun	1/2
Dried Bread Crumbs	3 Tbs.
Tortilla, 6"	1

Cereal

Bran Flakes	1/2 cup
Other ready-to-eat unsweetened Cereal	3/4 cup
Puffed Cereal (unfrosted)	1 cup
Cereal (cooked)	1/2 cup
Grits (cooked)	1/2 cup
Rice or Barley (cooked)	1/2 cup
Pasta (cooked), Spaghetti, Noodles, Macaroni	1/2 cup
Popcorn (popped, no fat added,large kernel)	3 cups
Cornmeal (dry)	2 Tbs.
Flour	2-1/2 Tbs.
Wheat Germ	1/4 cup

Crackers

Arrowroot	3
Graham, 2-1/2" sq.	2
Matzoth, 4" x 6"	1/2
Oyster	20

Pretzels, 3-1/8" long x 1/8" dia.	25	Prepared Foods	
Rye Wafers, 2" x 3-1/2"	3	Biscuit 2" dia.	1
Saltines	6	(omit 1 Fat Exchange)	
Soda, 2-1/2" sq.	4	Corn Bread, 2" x 2" x 1"	1

Dried Beans, Peas and Lentils

Corn Bread... (omit 1 Fat Exchange)
Corn Muffin, 2" dia. — 1

Beans, Peas, Lentils (dried and cooked)	1/2 cup	(omit 1 Fat Exchange)	
Baked Beans, no pork (canned)	1/4 cup	Crackers, round butter type (omit 1 Fat Exchange)	5
		Muffin, plain small	1

Starchy Vegetables

		(omit 1 Fat Exchange)	
Corn	1/3 cup	Potatoes, French Fried, length 2" to 3-1/2"	8
Corn on Cob	1 small	(omit 1 Fat Exchange)	
Lima Beans	1/2 cup	Potato or Corn Chips	15
Parsnips	2/3 cup	(omit 2 Fat Exchanges)	
Peas, Green (canned or frozen)	1/2 cup	Pancake, 5" x 1/2"	1
Potato, White	1 small	(omit 1 Fat Exchange)	
Potato (mashed)	1/2 cup	Waffle, 5" x 1/2"	1
Pumpkin	3/4 cup	(omit 1 Fat Exchange)	
Winter Squash, Acorn or Butternut	1/2 cup		
Yam or Sweet Potato	1/4 cup		

LIST 5 — Meat Exchanges
Lean Meat

One Exchange of Lean Meat (1 oz.) contains 7 grams of protein, 3 grams of fat and 55 calories.

All of the foods in the Meat Exchange Lists are good sources of protein and many are also good sources of iron, zinc, vitamin B_{12} (present only in foods of animal origin) and other vitamins of the vitamin B-complex.

Cholesterol is of animal origin. Foods of plant origin have no cholesterol.

Oysters are outstanding for their high content of zinc. Crab, liver, trimmed lean meats, the dark muscle meat of turkey, dried beans and peas and peanut butter all have much less zinc than oysters but are still good sources.

Dried beans, peas and peanut butter are particularly good sources of magnesium; also potassium. Your choice of meat groups through the week will depend on your blood lipid values. Consult with your diet counselor and your physician regarding your selection.

You may use the meat, fish or other Meat Exchanges that are prepared for the family when no fat or flour has been added. If meat is fried, use the fat included in the Meal Plan. Meat juices with the fat removed may be used with your meat or vegetables for added flavor. **Be certain to trim off all visible fat** and measure after it has been cooked. A three-ounce serving of cooked meat is about equal to four ounces of raw meat.

To plan a diet low in saturated fat and cholesterol, choose only those Exchanges in **bold type**.

This List shows the kinds and amounts of **Lean Meat** and other Protein-Rich Foods to use for one Low-Fat Meat Exchange. **Trim off all visible fat.**

Beef:	**Baby Beef (very lean), Chipped Beef, Chuck, Flank Steak, Tenderloin, Plate Ribs, Plate Skirt Steak, Round (bottom, top), All cuts Rump, Spare Ribs, Tripe**	1 oz.
Lamb:	**Leg, Rib, Sirloin, Loin (roast and chops), Shank, Shoulder**	1 oz.
Pork:	**Leg (Whole Rump, Center Shank), Ham, Smoked (center slices)**	1 oz.
Veal:	**Leg, Loin, Rib, Shank, Shoulder, Cutlets**	1 oz.

Poultry: Meat without skin **of Chicken, Turkey, Cornish Hen,**   1 oz.
         Guinea Hen, Pheasant
Fish: **Any fresh or frozen**   1 oz.
            Canned Salmon, Tuna, Mackerel, Crab and Lobster,   1/4 cup
            Clams, Oysters, Scallops, Shrimp,   5 or 1 oz.
            Sardines, drained   3
Cheeses containing less than 5% butterfat   1 oz.
Cottage Cheese, Dry and 2% butterfat   1/4 cup
Dried Beans and Peas (omit 1 Bread Exchange)   1/2 cup

LIST 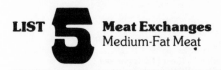 **Meat Exchanges**
Medium-Fat Meat

One Exhange of Medium-Fat
Meat (1 oz.) contains 7 grams of
protein, 5 grams of fat and
75 calories.

This List shows the kinds and amounts of Medium-Fat Meat and other Protein-Rich
Foods to use for one Medium-Fat Meat Exchange. **Trim off all visible fat.**

Beef: Ground (15% fat), Corned Beef (canned), Rib Eye, Round   1 oz.
           (ground commercial)
Pork: Loin (all cuts Tenderloin), Shoulder Arm (picnic), Shoulder Blade,   1 oz.
           Boston Butt, Canadian Bacon, Boiled Ham
Liver, Heart, Kidney and Sweetbreads (these are high in cholesterol)   1 oz.
Cottage Cheese, creamed   1/4 cup
Cheese: Mozzarella, Ricotta, Farmer's cheese, Neufchatel,   1 oz.
          Parmesan   3 tbs.
Egg (high in cholesterol)   1
Peanut Butter (omit 2 additional Fat Exchanges)   2 tbs.

LIST 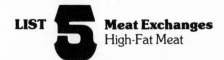 **Meat Exchanges**
High-Fat Meat

One Exchange of High-Fat Meat
(1 oz.) contains 7 grams of protein,
8 grams of fat and 100 calories.

This List shows the kinds and amounts of High-Fat Meat and other Protein-Rich Foods
to use for one High-Fat Meat Exchange. **Trim off all visible fat.**

Beef: Brisket, Corned Beef (Brisket), Ground Beef (more than   1 oz.
           20% fat), Hamburger (commercial), Chuck (ground
           commercial), Roasts (Rib), Steaks (Club and Rib)
Lamb: Breast   1 oz.
Pork: Spare Ribs, Loin (Back Ribs), Pork (ground), Country style   1 oz.
           Ham, Deviled Ham
Veal: Breast   1 oz.
Poultry: Capon, Duck (domestic), Goose   1 oz.
Cheese: Cheddar Types   1 oz.
Cold Cuts   4-1/2"x 1/8" slice
Frankfurter   1 small

LIST 6   **Fat Exchanges**   One Exchange of Fat contains 5 grams of fat and 45 calories.

Fats are of both animal and vegetable origin and range from liquid oils to hard fats. Oils are fats that remain liquid at room temperature and are usually of vegetable origin. Common fats obtained from vegetables are corn oil, olive oil and peanut oil. Some of the common animal fats are butter and bacon fat.

Since all fats are concentrated sources of calories, foods on this List should be measured carefully to control weight. Margarine, butter, cream and cream cheese contain vitamin A. Use the fats on this List in the amounts on the Meal Plan.

This List shows the kinds and amounts of Fat-Containing Foods to use for one Fat Exchange. To plan a diet low in Saturated Fat select only those Exchanges which appear in **bold type**. They are **Polyunsaturated.**

Margarine, soft, tub or stick*	1 teaspoon
Avocado (4″ in diameter)**	1/8
Oil, Corn, Cottonseed, Safflower,	
Soy, Sunflower	1 teaspoon
Oil, Olive**	1 teaspoon
Oil, Peanut**	1 teaspoon
Olives**	5 small
Almonds**	10 whole
Pecans**	2 large whole
Peanuts**	
Spanish	20 whole
Virginia	10 whole
Walnuts	6 small
Nuts, other**	6 small
Margarine, regular stick	1 teaspoon
Butter	1 teaspoon
Bacon fat	1 teaspoon
Bacon, crisp	1 strip
Cream, light	2 tablespoons
Cream, sour	2 tablespoons
Cream, heavy	1 tablespoon
Cream Cheese	1 tablespoon
French dressing***	1 tablespoon
Italian dressing***	1 tablespoon
Lard	1 teaspoon
Mayonnaise***	1 teaspoon
Salad dressing, mayonnaise type***	2 teaspoons
Salt pork	3/4 inch cube

  *Made with corn, cottonseed, safflower, soy or sunflower oil only
 **Fat content is primarily monounsaturated
***If made with corn, cottonseed, safflower, soy or sunflower oil
   can be used on fat modified diet

Index